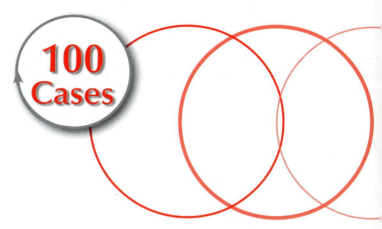

100 Cases

in Clinical
Medicine
Third edition

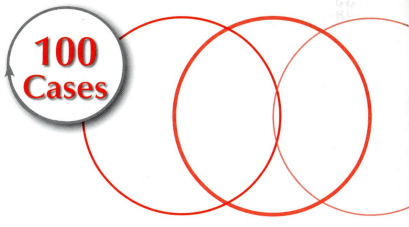

in Clinical
Medicine
Third edition

P John Rees MB BChir MD FRCP FRCPE FKC
Professor of Medical Education,
King's College London School of Medicine at Guy's,
King's and St Thomas' Hospitals, London, UK

James Pattison MA DM FRCP
Consultant Nephrologist,
Guy's and St Thomas' NHS Foundation Trust,
London, UK

Christopher Kosky MBBS FRACP
Consultant Physician,
General and Respiratory Medicine & Sleep Disorders,
Guy's and St Thomas' NHS Foundation Trust;
Honorary Senior Lecturer, King's College London, UK

100 Cases Series Editor:

Janice Rymer MD FRCOG FRANZCOG FHEA
Dean of Undergraduate Medicine and Professor of Gynaecology,
King's College London School of Medicine, London, UK

CRC Press
Taylor & Francis Group
Boca Raton London New York

CRC Press is an imprint of the
Taylor & Francis Group, an **informa** business

CRC Press
Taylor & Francis Group
6000 Broken Sound Parkway NW, Suite 300
Boca Raton, FL 33487-2742

© 2014 by Taylor & Francis Group, LLC
CRC Press is an imprint of Taylor & Francis Group, an Informa business

No claim to original U.S. Government works

Printed on acid-free paper
Version Date: 20130808

Printed and bound in India by Replika Press Pvt. Ltd.

International Standard Book Number-13: 978-1-4441-7429-8 (Paperback)

Visit the Taylor & Francis Web site at
http://www.taylorandfrancis.com

and the CRC Press Web site at
http://www.crcpress.com

#8723G3981

CONTENTS

PREFACE

Most doctors think that the most memorable way to learn medicine is to see patients. It is easier to recall information based on a real person than a page in a textbook. Another important element in the retention of information is the depth of learning. Learning that seeks to understand problems is more likely to be accessible later than superficial factual accumulation. This is the basis of problem-based learning, whereby students explore problems with the help of a facilitator. The cases in this book are designed to provide another useful approach, parallel to seeing patients and giving an opportunity for self-directed exploration of clinical problems. They are based on the findings of history taking and examination, together with the need to evaluate initial investigations such as blood investigations, X-rays and electrocardiograms.

These cases are no substitute for clinical experience with real patients, but they provide a safe environment for students to explore clinical problems and their own approach to diagnosis and management. Most are common problems that might present to a general practitioner's surgery, a medical outpatients clinic or a session on call in hospital. There are a few more unusual cases to illustrate specific points and to emphasize that rare things do present, even if they are uncommon. The cases are written to try to interest students in clinical problems and to enthuse them to find out more. They try to explore thinking about diagnosis and management of real clinical situations.

The first 20 cases are arranged by systems, but the next 80 are in random order since, in medicine, symptoms such as breathlessness and pain may relate to many different clinical problems in various systems. We hope you enjoy working through the problems presented here and can put the lessons you learn into practice in your student days and subsequent career.

P John Rees
James Pattison
Gwyn Williams

ACKNOWLEDGEMENTS

The authors would like to thank the following people for their help with illustrations Dr A Saunders, Dr S Rankin, Dr J Reidy, Dr J Bingham, Dr L Macdonald, Dr G Cook, Dr T Gibson, Professor R Reznak, Dr B Lams, Dr J Chambers, Dr H Milburn and Dr J Gilmore.

ABBREVIATIONS

AAT	alanine aminotransferase
ACE	angiotensin-converting enzyme
ACTH	adrenocorticotrophic hormone
ADH	antidiuretic hormone
ADPKD	autosomal dominant polycystic kidney disease
APTT	activated partial thromboplastin time ·
ARAS	atherosclerotic renal artery stenosis
AVP	arginine vasopressin
BCG	bacille Calmette–Guérin
BMI	body mass index
CJD	Creutzfeldt–Jakob disease
CMV	cytomegalovirus
COPD	chronic obstructive pulmonary disease
CRP	C-reactive protein
CSF	cerebrospinal fluid
CT	computed tomography
CVP	central venous pressure
DDAVP	I-deamino-8-d-arginine vasopressin
DEXA	dual-energy X-ray absorptiometry
DOT	directly observed therapy
DVT	deep vein thrombosis
EBV	Epstein–Barr virus
ECG	electrocardiogram
EEG	electroencephalogram
EMG	electromyogram
ERCP	endoscopic retrograde cholangiopancreatography
ESR	erythrocyte sedimentation rate
FER	forced expiratory ratio
FEV_1	forced expiratory volume in 1 s
FMD	fibromuscular dysplasia
FSH	follicle-stimulating hormone
FVC	forced vital capacity
GnRH	gonadotrophin-releasing hormone
GP	general practitioner
HbA_{1c}	haemoglobin A_{1c}
HDL	high-density lipoprotein
5-HIAA	5-hydroxyindole acetic acid
5-HT	5-hydroxytryptamine
IBS	irritable bowel syndrome
ICU	intensive care unit
IgG	immunoglobulin G
IgM	immunoglobulin M
INR	international normalized ratio
IPF	idiopathic pulmonary fibrosis
ITP	idiopathic thrombocytopenic purpura
JVP	jugular venous pressure
LDL	low-density lipoprotein
LH	luteinizing hormone
MCV	mean corpuscular volume
MRSA	methicillin-resistant *Staphylococcus aureus*
NAD	nothing abnormal detected

NGU	non-gonococcal urethritis
NSAID	non-steroidal anti-inflammatory drug
NSIP	non-specific interstitial pneumonitis
nvCJD	new-variant CJD
$PaCO_2$	arterial partial pressure of carbon dioxide
pco_2	partial pressure of carbon dioxide
PEF	peak expiratory flow
PET	positron-emission tomography
po_2	partial pressure of oxygen
SIADH	syndrome of inappropriate ADH secretion
SLE	systemic lupus erythematosus
STD	sexually transmitted diseases
T4	thyroxine
TIA	transient ischaemic attack
TIBC	total iron-binding capacity
TNF	tissue necrosis factor
TSH	thyroid-stimulating hormone
TTP	thrombotic thrombocytopenic purpura
UIP	usual interstitial pneumonia
VDRL	venereal disease research laboratory
VLDL	very low-density lipoprotein
WOSCOPS	West of Scotland Coronary Prevention Study

Section 1

SYSTEMS-RELATED CASES

CARDIOLOGY

CASE 1: DIZZINESS

History

A 75-year-old man is brought to hospital with an episode of dizziness. He still feels unwell when he is seen 30 min after the onset. He was well until 6 months ago and then started having falls. On some occasions the falls have been associated with loss of consciousness, although he is unsure of the length of time he was unconscious. On other occasions he has felt dizzy and has had to sit down, but has not lost consciousness. These episodes usually happened on exertion, but once or twice they have occurred while sitting down. He recovers over 10–15 min after each episode.

He lives alone, and most of the episodes have not been witnessed. Once his granddaughter was with him when he blacked out. Worried, she called an ambulance. He looked so pale and still that she thought that he had died. He was taken to hospital, by which time he had recovered completely and was discharged and told that he had a normal electrocardiogram (ECG) and chest X-ray.

There is no history of chest pain or palpitations. He has had gout and some urinary frequency. A diagnosis of benign prostatic hypertrophy has been made, for which he is on no treatment. He takes ibuprofen occasionally for the gout. He stopped smoking 5 years ago. He drinks 5–10 units of alcohol weekly. The dizziness and blackouts have not been associated with alcohol. There is no relevant family history. He used to work as an electrician.

Examination

He is pale with a blood pressure of 96/64 mmHg. The pulse rate is 33/min, regular. There are no heart murmurs. The jugular venous pressure is raised 3 cm with occasional rises. There is no leg oedema; the peripheral pulses are palpable except for the left dorsalis pedis. The respiratory system is normal.

🔍 INVESTIGATIONS

- The patient's ECG is shown in Figure 1.1.

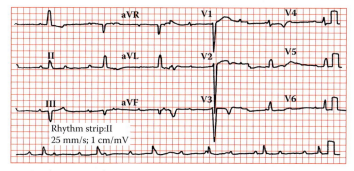

Figure 1.1 Patient's electrocardiogram.

Questions

- What is the cause of his blackout?
- What does the ECG show?

ANSWER 1

The blackouts do not seem to have had any relationship to posture. They have been a mixture of dizziness and loss of consciousness. The one witnessed episode seems to have been associated with loss of colour. This suggests a loss of cardiac output usually associated with an arrhythmia. This may be the case despite the absence of any other cardiac symptoms. There may be an obvious flushing of the skin as cardiac output and blood flow return.

The normal ECG and chest X-ray when he attended hospital after an episode do not rule out an intermittent conduction problem. On this occasion the symptoms have remained in a more minor form. The ECG shows third-degree or complete heart block (Figure 1.2). There is complete dissociation of the atrial rate and the ventricular rate, which is 33/min. The episodes of loss of consciousness are called Stokes–Adams attacks and are caused by self-limited rapid tachyarrhythmias at the onset of heart block or transient asystole. Although these have been intermittent in the past, he is now in stable complete heart block, and if this continues, the slow ventricular rate will be associated with reduced cardiac output, which may cause fatigue, dizziness on exertion or heart failure. Intermittent failure of the escape rhythm may cause syncope.

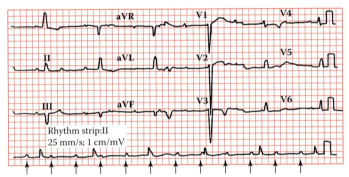

Figure 1.2 Electrocardiogram showing complete heart block, p-waves arrowed.

On examination, the occasional rises in the jugular venous pressure are intermittent 'cannon' a-waves as the right atrium contracts against a closed tricuspid valve. In addition, the intensity of the first heart sound will vary.

> **! Differential diagnosis**
>
> The differential diagnosis of transient loss of consciousness splits into neurological and vascular causes. A witness is very helpful in differentiation. Neurological causes are various forms of epilepsy, often with associated features. Vascular causes are related to local or general reduction in cerebral blood flow. Local reduction may occur in transient ischaemic attacks or vertebrobasilar insufficiency. A more global reduction, often with pallor, occurs with arrhythmias, postural hypotension and vasovagal faints.

The treatment should be insertion of a pacemaker. If the rhythm in complete heart block is stable, then a permanent pacemaker should be inserted as soon as this can be arranged. This should be a dual-chamber system pacing the atria, then the ventricles (DDD, dual sensing and pacing, triggered by atrial sensing, inhibited by ventricular sensing) or possibly a ventricular pacing system (VVI, pacing the ventricle, inhibited by ventricular sensing). If there is doubt about the ventricular escape rhythm, then a temporary pacemaker should be inserted immediately.

KEY POINTS

- When a patient suffers transient loss of consciousness, a careful history from a witness may help with the diagnosis.
- Normal examination and ECG do not rule out intermittent serious arrhythmias.
- Large waves in the jugular venous pressure are usually regular giant v-waves in tricuspid regurgitation or intermittent cannon a-waves in complete heart block.

CASE 2: CHEST PAIN

History

A 34-year-old male accountant comes to the emergency department with acute chest pain. There is a previous history of occasional stabbing chest pain for 2 years. The current pain had come on 4h earlier at 8pm and has been persistent since then. It is central in position, with some radiation to both sides of the chest. It is not associated with shortness of breath or palpitations. The pain is relieved by sitting up and leaning forward. Two paracetamol tablets taken earlier at 9pm did not make any difference to the pain.

The previous chest pain had been occasional, lasting a second or two at a time and with no particular precipitating factors. It has usually been on the left side of the chest, although the position had varied.

Two weeks previously he had an upper respiratory tract infection that lasted 4 days. This consisted of a sore throat, blocked nose, sneezing and a cough. His wife and two children were ill at the same time with similar symptoms but have been well since then. He has a history of migraine. In the family history his father had a myocardial infarction at the age of 51 years and was found to have a marginally high cholesterol level. His mother and two sisters, aged 36 and 38 years, are well. After his father's infarct the accountant had his lipids measured; cholesterol was 5.1 mmol/L (desirable range, 5.5 mmol/L). He is a non-smoker who drinks 15 units of alcohol per week.

Examination

His pulse rate is 75/min, blood pressure 124/78 mmHg. His temperature is 37.8°C. There is nothing abnormal to find in the cardiovascular and respiratory systems.

🔍 **INVESTIGATIONS**

- A chest X-ray is normal. The haemoglobin and white cell count are normal. ESR 46. The troponin level is slightly raised. Other biochemical tests are normal.
- The electrocardiogram (ECG) is shown in Figure 2.1.

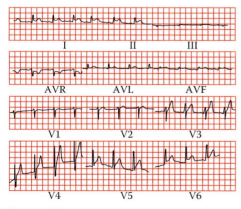

Figure 2.1 Electrocardiogram.

Question

- What is the diagnosis?

ANSWER 2

The previous chest pains lasting a second or two are unlikely to be of any real significance. Cardiac pain, and virtually any other significant pain, lasts longer than this, and stabbing momentary left-sided chest pains are quite common. The positive family history increases the risk of ischaemic heart disease, but there are no other risk factors evident from the history and examination. Chest pain due to pericarditis is usually sharp and pleuritic, and exacerbated by inspiration or coughing. The relief from sitting up and leaning forward is typical of pain originating in the pericardium. The ECG shows elevation of the ST segment, which is concave upwards, typical of pericarditis and unlike the upward convexity found in the ST elevation after myocardial infarction. ST changes are typically present in most leads in acute pericarditis, unlike the changes in myocardial infarction which are limited to anatomical groupings of leads that correspond to the area of the infarct.

The story of an upper respiratory tract infection shortly before suggests that this may well have a viral aetiology. The viruses commonly involved in pericarditis are Coxsackie B viruses. The absence of a pericardial rub does not rule out pericarditis. Rubs often vary in intensity and may not always be audible. If this diagnosis was suspected, it is often worth listening again on a number of occasions for the rub. Pericardial rubs have a scratchy quality that is best heard with the diaphragm of the stethoscope. Pericarditis often involves some adjacent myocardial inflammation, and this could explain the rise in troponin levels. As pericarditis is an inflammatory disease, the white cell count, ESR and serum CRP are often raised. Echocardiography often shows a small pericardial effusion, with tamponade being rare.

Pericarditis may occur as a complication of a myocardial infarction, but this tends to occur a day or more later—inflammation either as a direct result of death of the underlying heart muscle or as a later immunological effect (Dressler's syndrome). Pericarditis also occurs as part of various connective tissue disorders, tuberculosis, uraemia and involvement from other local infections or tumours. Myocardial infarction is not common at the age of 34 years, but it certainly occurs. Other causes of chest pain, such as oesophageal pain or musculoskeletal pain, are not suggested by the history and investigations.

A subsequent rise in antibody titres against Coxsackie virus suggested a viral pericarditis. Symptoms and ECG changes resolved in 4–5 days. An echocardiogram showed a small pericardial effusion and good left ventricular muscle function. The symptoms settled with rest and non-steroidal anti-inflammatory drugs.

 KEY POINTS

- ST segment elevation that is concave upwards is characteristic of pericarditis.
- Viral pericarditis in young people is most often caused by Coxsackie viruses.
- Myocarditis may be associated with pericarditis, and muscle function should be assessed on echocardiogram and damage assessed from troponin measurements.

RESPIRATORY

CASE 3: CHRONIC COUGH

History

A 19-year-old boy has a history of repeated chest infections. He had problems with a cough and sputum production in the first 2 years of life and was labelled as bronchitic. Over the next 14 years he was often 'chesty' and had spent 4–5 weeks a year away from school. Over the past 2 years he has developed more problems and was admitted to hospital on three occasions with cough and purulent sputum. On the first two occasions, *Haemophilus influenzae* was grown on culture of the sputum, and on the last occasion 2 months previously, *Pseudomonas aeruginosa* was isolated from the sputum at the time of admission to hospital. He is still coughing up sputum. Although he has largely recovered from the infection, his mother is worried and asked for a further sputum sample to be sent off. The report has come back from the microbiology laboratory showing that there is a scanty growth of *Pseudomonas* on culture of the sputum.

There is no family history of any chest disease. Routine questioning shows that his appetite is reasonable, micturition is normal and his bowels tend to be irregular.

Examination

On examination he is thin, weighing 48 kg, and is 1.6 m (5 ft 6 in) tall.

- The only finding in the chest is of a few inspiratory crackles over the upper zones of both lungs. Cardiovascular and abdominal examination is normal.

🔍 INVESTIGATIONS

- The chest X-ray is shown in Figure 3.1.

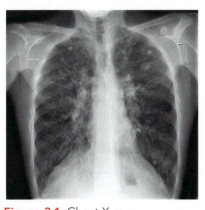

Figure 3.1 Chest X-ray.

Questions

- What does the X-ray show?
- What is the most likely diagnosis?
- What investigations should be performed?

ANSWER 3

The chest X-ray shows abnormal shadowing throughout both lungs, more marked in both upper lobes, with some ring shadows and tubular shadows representing thickened bronchial walls. These findings would be compatible with a diagnosis of bronchiectasis. The pulmonary arteries are prominent, suggesting a degree of pulmonary hypertension. The distribution is typical of that found in cystic fibrosis, where the changes are most evident in the upper lobes. Most other forms of bronchiectasis are more likely to occur in the lower lobes, where drainage by gravity is less effective. High-resolution computed tomography (CT) of the lungs is the best way to diagnose bronchiectasis and to define its extent and distribution. In younger and milder cases of cystic fibrosis, the predominant organisms in the sputum are *Haemophilus influenzae* and *Staphylococcus aureus*. Later, as more lung damage occurs, *Pseudomonas aeruginosa* is a common pathogen. Once present in the lungs in cystic fibrosis, it is difficult or impossible to remove it completely.

Cystic fibrosis should always be considered when there is a story of repeated chest infections in a young person. Although it presents most often below the age of 20 years, diagnosis may be delayed until the 20s, 30s, 40s or later in milder cases. Associated problems occur in the pancreas (malabsorption, diabetes), sinuses and liver. It has become evident that some patients are affected more mildly, especially those with the less-common genetic variants. These milder cases may only be affected by the chest problems of cystic fibrosis and have little or no malabsorption from the pancreatic insufficiency.

> **! Differential diagnosis**
>
> The differential diagnosis in this young man would be other causes of diffuse bronchiectasis, such as agammaglobulinaemia or immotile cilia. Respiratory function should be measured to see the degree of functional impairment. Bronchiectasis in the upper lobes may occur in tuberculosis or in allergic bronchopulmonary aspergillosis associated with asthma.

The common diagnostic test for cystic fibrosis is to measure the electrolytes in the sweat, where there is an abnormally high concentration of sodium and chloride. At the age of 19 years, the sweat test may be less reliable. It is more specific if repeated after the administration of fludrocortisone. An alternative would be to have the potential difference across the nasal epithelium measured at a centre with a special interest in cystic fibrosis. Cystic fibrosis has an autosomal recessive inheritance with the commonest genetic abnormality ΔF508 found in 85 per cent of cases. The gene is responsible for the protein controlling chloride transport across the cell membrane. The commoner genetic abnormalities can be identified, and the current battery of genetic tests identifies well over 95 per cent of cases. However, the absence of ΔF508 and other common abnormalities would not rule out cystic fibrosis related to the less-common genetic variants.

In later stages, lung transplantation can be considered. Since the identification of the genetic abnormality, trials of gene-replacement therapy have begun.

Management should be at a centre with experience in the management of adult cystic fibrosis. Treatment at such centres for children, adolescents and adults is associated with improved outcomes.

KEY POINTS

- Milder forms of cystic fibrosis may present in adolescence and adulthood.
- Milder forms are often related to less-common genetic abnormalities.
- A high-resolution CT scan is the best way to detect bronchiectasis and to define its extent.
- Management should be at an experienced cystic fibrosis centre.

CASE 4: SHORTNESS OF BREATH

History

A 26-year-old teacher has consulted her general practitioner (GP) for her persistent cough. She wants to have a second course of antibiotics because an initial course of amoxicillin made no difference. The cough has troubled her for 3 months, since she moved to a new school. The cough is now disturbing her sleep and making her tired during the day. She teaches games, and the cough is troublesome when going out to the playground and when jogging. In her medical history she had her appendix removed 3 years ago. She had her tonsils removed as a child and was said to have recurrent episodes of bronchitis between the ages of 3 and 6 years. She has never smoked and takes no medication other than an oral contraceptive. Her parents are alive, and well and she has two brothers, one of whom has hay fever.

Examination

The respiratory rate is 18/min. Her chest is clear, and there are no abnormalities in the nose or pharynx or the cardiovascular, respiratory or nervous systems.

🔍 INVESTIGATIONS

- Chest X-ray is reported as normal.
- Spirometry is carried out at the surgery, and she is asked to record her peak flow rate at home, the best of three readings every morning and every evening for 2 weeks. Spirometry results are as follows:

	Actual	Predicted
FEV$_1$ (L)	3.9	3.6–4.2
FVC (L)	5.0	4.5–5.4
FER (FEV$_1$/FVC) (%)	78	75–80
PEF (L/min)	470	440–540

FEV$_1$: forced expiratory volume in 1 s; FVC, forced vital capacity; FER, forced expiratory ratio; PEF, peak expiratory flow.

A peak flow recording is shown in Figure 4.1.

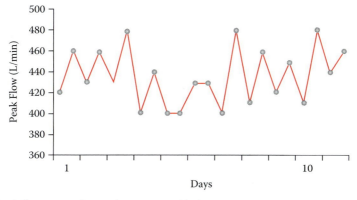

Figure 4.1 Peak flow recording at home over 11 days.

Questions

- What is your interpretation of these findings?
- What do you think is the likely diagnosis, and what would be appropriate treatment?

ANSWER 4

The peak flow pattern shows a degree of diurnal variation. This does not reach the diagnostic criteria for asthma, but it is suspicious. The mean daily variation in peak flow from the recordings is 36 L/min, and the mean evening peak flow is 453 L/min, giving a mean diurnal variation of 8 per cent. There is a small diurnal variation in normals, and a variation of >15 per cent is diagnostic of asthma. In this patient the label of 'bronchitis' as a child was probably asthma. The family history of an atopic condition (hay fever in a brother) and the triggering of the cough by exercise and going out in the cold also suggest bronchial hyper-responsiveness typical of asthma.

Patients with a chronic persistent cough of unexplained cause should have a chest X-ray. When the X-ray is clear the cough is likely to be produced by one of three main causes in non-smokers. Around half of such cases have asthma or will go on to develop asthma over the next few years. Half of the rest have rhinitis or sinusitis with a postnasal drip. In around 20 per cent the cough is related to gastro-oesophageal reflux. A small number of cases will be caused by otherwise-unsuspected problems such as foreign bodies, bronchial 'adenoma', sarcoidosis or fibrosing alveolitis. Cough is a common side effect in patients treated with angiotensin-converting enzyme (ACE) inhibitors.

In this patient the diagnosis of asthma was confirmed with an exercise test, which was associated with a 25 per cent drop in FEV after completion of 6 min of vigorous exercise. Alternative bronchoprovocation tests include the use of inhaled methacholine or histamine, and a fall in FEV_1 greater than 20 per cent.

After the exercise test, an inhaled steroid was given, and the cough settled after 1 week. The inhaled steroid was discontinued after 4 weeks and replaced by a β_2-agonist to use before exercise. However, the cough recurred with more evident wheeze and shortness of breath, and treatment was changed back to an inhaled steroid with a β_2-agonist as needed. If control was not established, the next step would be to check inhaler technique and treatment adherence and to consider adding a long-acting β_2-agonist. In some cases, the persistent dry cough associated with asthma may require more vigorous treatment than this. Inhaled steroids for a month or more or even a 2-week course of oral steroids may be needed to relieve the cough. The successful management of dry cough relies on establishing the correct diagnosis and treating it vigorously.

 KEY POINTS

- The three commonest causes of persistent dry cough with a normal chest X-ray are asthma (50 per cent), sinusitis and postnasal drip (25 per cent) and reflux oesophagitis (20 per cent).
- Asthma may present as a cough (cough-variant asthma) with little or no airflow obstruction initially, although this develops later.
- Persistent cough with normal chest examination is unlikely to have a bacterial cause or respond to antibiotic treatment.

ABDOMEN

CASE 5: ACUTE ABDOMINAL PAIN

History

A 56-year-old woman presents to the emergency department complaining of abdominal pain. Twenty-four hours previously she developed a continuous pain in the upper abdomen that has become progressively more severe. The pain radiates into the back. She feels nauseated and alternately hot and cold. Her past medical history is notable for a duodenal ulcer, which was successfully treated with *Helicobacter* eradication therapy 5 years earlier. She smokes 15 cigarettes a day and shares a bottle of wine each evening with her husband.

Examination

The patient looks unwell and dehydrated. She weighs 115 kg. She is febrile, 38.5°C; her pulse is 108/min, and blood pressure is 124/76 mmHg. Cardiovascular and respiratory system examination is normal. She is tender in the right upper quadrant and epigastrium, with guarding and rebound tenderness. Bowel sounds are sparse.

INVESTIGATIONS		
		Normal
Haemoglobin	14.7 g/dL	11.7–15.7 g/dL
White cell count	19.8 × 10⁹/L	3.5–11.0 × 10⁹/L
Platelets	239 × 10⁹/L	150–440 × 10⁹/L
Sodium	137 mmol/L	135–145 mmol/L
Potassium	4.8 mmol/L	3.5–5.0 mmol/L
Urea	8.6 mmol/L	2.5–6.7 mmol/L
Creatinine	116 µmol/L	70–120 µmol/L
Bilirubin	19 µmol/L	3–17 µmol/L
Alkaline phosphatase	58 IU/L	30–300 IU/L
Alanine aminotransferase (AAT)	67 IU/L	5–35 IU/L
Gamma-glutamyl transpeptidase	72 IU/L	11–51 IU/L
C-reactive protein (CRP)	256 mg/L	<5 mg/L

A plain abdominal X-ray is shown in Figure 5.1.

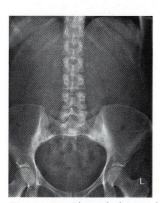

Figure 5.1 Plain abdominal X-ray.

Questions

- What is the most likely diagnosis?
- How would you manage this patient?

ANSWER 5

This woman has acute cholecystitis. Cholecystitis is most common in obese, middle-aged women and classically is triggered by eating a fatty meal. Cholecystitis is usually caused by a gallstone impacting in the cystic duct. Continued secretion by the gallbladder leads to increased pressure and inflammation of the gallbladder wall. Bacterial infection is usually by Gram-negative organisms and anaerobes. Ischaemia in the distended gallbladder can lead to perforation, causing either generalized peritonitis or formation of a localized abscess. Alternatively the stone can spontaneously disimpact and the symptoms spontaneously improve. Gallstones can become stuck in the common bile duct, leading to cholangitis or pancreatitis. Rarely, gallstones can perforate through the inflamed gallbladder wall into the small intestine and cause intestinal obstruction (gallstone ileus).

The typical symptom of acute cholecystitis is sudden-onset right upper quadrant abdominal pain that radiates into the back. An episode of prolonged right upper quadrant pain associated with fever, suggests acute cholecystits rather than simple biliary colic. Jaundice usually occurs if there is a stone in the common bile duct.

There is usually fever, tachycardia, guarding and rebound tenderness in the right upper quadrant (Murphy's sign). In this patient the leucocytosis and raised CRP are consistent with acute cholecystitis. If the serum bilirubin and liver enzymes are very deranged, acute cholangitis due to a stone in the common bile duct should be suspected. The abdominal X-ray is normal; the majority of gallstones are radiolucent and do not show on plain films.

> **! Differential diagnosis**
>
> The major differential diagnoses of acute cholecystitis include biliary colic, perforated peptic ulcer, acute pancreatitis, acute hepatitis, subphrenic abscess, retrocaecal appendicitis, right pyelonephritis and perforated carcinoma or diverticulum of the hepatic flexure of the colon. Myocardial infarction or right lower lobe pneumonia may also mimic cholecystitis.

This patient should be admitted under the surgical team. Serum amylase should be measured to rule out pancreatitis. Blood cultures should be taken. Chest X-ray should be performed to exclude pneumonia and erect abdominal X-ray to rule out air under the diaphragm, which occurs with a perforated peptic ulcer. An abdominal ultrasound will show gallstones and inflammation of the gallbladder wall. The patient should be kept nil by mouth, given intravenous fluids, analgesia and commenced on intravenous cephalosporins and metronidazole. The patient should be examined regularly for signs of generalized peritonitis or cholangitis. If the symptoms settle down the patient is normally discharged to be readmitted in a few weeks once the inflammation has settled down to have a cholecystectomy. There is a trend to performing immediate cholecystectomy in low risk patients.

> **🔑 KEY POINTS**
>
> - Acute cholecystitis typically causes right upper quadrant pain and a positive Murphy's sign.
> - Potential complications include septicaemia and peritonitis.

History

A 66-year-old woman, a retired nurse, consults her general practitioner (GP) with a 4-month history of tiredness, slight breathlessness on exertion and loss of weight from 71 to 65 kg. Her appetite is unchanged and normal; she has no nausea or vomiting, but over the last 2 months she has had an altered bowel habit with constipation alternating with her usual and normal pattern. She has not seen any blood in her faeces and has had no abdominal pain. She has had no post-menopausal bleeding. There is no relevant past or family history, and she is on no medication.

She has smoked 20 cigarettes daily for 48 years and drinks 20–28 units of alcohol a week.

Examination

She has slight pallor but otherwise looks well. No lymphadenopathy is detected, and her breasts, thyroid, heart, chest and abdomen, including rectal examination, are all normal. The blood pressure is 148/90 mmHg.

INVESTIGATIONS

		Normal
Haemoglobin	10.1 g/dL	11.7–15.7 g/dL
Mean corpuscular volume (MCV)	76 fL	80–99 fL
White cell count	4.9 × 10⁹/L	3.5–11.0 × 10⁹/L
Platelets	277 × 10⁹/L	150–440 × 10⁹/L
Sodium	142 mmol/L	135–145 mmol/L
Potassium	4.4 mmol/L	3.5–5.0 mmol/L
Urea	5.2 mmol/L	2.5–6.7 mmol/L
Creatinine	106 µmol/L	70–120 µmol/L

Urinalysis: no protein, no blood
Blood film shows a microcytic hypochromic picture.

Questions

- What is the likeliest diagnosis?
- How would you investigate the patient?

ANSWER 6

The investigations show a microcytic, hypochromic anaemia. In a premenopausal woman the most likely cause would be excessive menstrual blood loss. In men or postmenopausal women the most likely cause would be loss from the gastrointestinal tract. This woman has an altered bowel habit, which suggests a problem with the lower gastrointestinal tract and a diagnosis of carcinoma of the colon, which would also explain her weight loss. A barium enema revealed a neoplasm in the sigmoid colon, confirmed by colonoscopy and biopsy. Chest X-ray and abdominal ultrasound showed no pulmonary metastases and no intra-abdominal lymphadenopathy or hepatic metastases, respectively.

She proceeded to a sigmoid colectomy and end-to-end anastomosis and was regularly followed-up for any evidence of recurrence. Histology showed a grade I tumour.

Carcinoma of the colon is increasing in frequency. If it presents at an early stage, then the prospect for cure is good. Rectal bleeding, alteration in bowel habit for longer than 1 month at any age, or iron-deficient anaemia in men or postmenopausal women are indications for investigation of the gastrointestinal tract. In younger people there may be a hereditary element to carcinoma of the colon.

Smoking is a risk factor for carcinoma of the colon.

 KEY POINTS

- Carcinoma of the colon can present with few or no symptoms or signs in the gastrointestinal tract.
- Unexplained iron deficiency anaemia warrants investigation of the upper and lower gastrointestinal tract.

LIVER

History

A man of 45 consults his general practitioner (GP) with a 6-month history of reduced appetite and weight loss, from 78 to 71 kg. During the last 3 months he has had intermittent nausea, especially in the mornings, and in the last 3 months the morning nausea has been accompanied by vomiting on several occasions. For 1 month he has noted swelling of his ankles. Despite his weight loss he has recently noticed his trousers getting tighter. He has had no abdominal pain. He has no relevant past history and knows no family history as he was adopted. He takes no medication. From the age of 18 he has smoked 5–6 cigarettes daily and drunk 15–20 units of alcohol per week. He has been a chef all his working life, without exception in fashionable restaurants. He now lives alone as his wife left him 1 year ago.

Examination

He has plethoric features. There is pitting oedema of his ankles. He appears to have lost weight from his limbs, but not his trunk. He has nine spider naevi on his upper trunk. His pulse is normal, and the rate is 92/min. His jugular venous pressure (JVP) is not raised, and his blood pressure is 146/84 mmHg. The cardiovascular and respiratory systems are normal. The abdomen is distended. He has no palpable masses, but there is shifting dullness and a fluid thrill.

INVESTIGATIONS

		Normal
Haemoglobin	12.6 g/dL	13.3–17.7 g/dL
Mean corpuscular volume (MCV)	107 fL	80–99 fL
White cell count	10.2×10^9/L	$3.9–10.6 \times 10^9$/L
Platelets	121×10^9/L	$150–440 \times 10^9$/L
Sodium	131 mmol/L	135–145 mmol/L
Potassium	4.2 mmol/L	3.5–5.0 mmol/L
Urea	2.2 mmol/L	2.5–6.7 mmol/L
Creatinine	101 μmol/L	70–120 μmol/L
Calcium	2.44 mmol/L	2.12–2.65 mmol/L
Phosphate	1.2 mmol/L	0.8–1.45 mmol/L
Total protein	48 g/L	60–80 g/L
Albumin	26 g/L	35–50 g/L
Bilirubin	25 mmol/L	3–17 mmol/L
Alanine transaminase	276 IU/L	5–35 IU/L
Gamma-glutamyl transaminase	873 IU/L	11–51 IU/L
Alkaline phosphatase	351 IU/L	30–300 IU/L
International normalised ratio (INR)	1.4	0.9–1.2

Urinalysis: no protein; no blood

Questions
- What is the diagnosis?
- How would you manage this patient?

ANSWER 7

This man has signs of chronic liver disease with ascites and oedema. The number of spider naevi is more than the accepted normal of three. The most common cause of chronic liver disease is alcohol. He is at increased risk of alcohol misuse because he works in the catering business. His symptoms of morning nausea and vomiting are typical of alcohol misuse. Chronic alcohol excess would account for his cushingoid appearance due to the increases of adrenocorticotrophic hormone [ACTH] secretion). Macrocytic anaemia can be due to dietary folate deficiency or the direct toxic action of alcohol on the bone marrow. The rise in bilirubin is insufficient to cause jaundice. The low serum albumin and raised international normalised ratio (INR) may be due to impaired synthetic function of clotting factors produced by the liver. Thrombocytopenia may be from platelet sequestration in an enlarged spleen as a result of portal hypertension from liver cirrhosis.

However, his alcohol intake is too low to be consistent with the diagnosis of alcoholic liver disease. When the provisional diagnosis is discussed with him, though, he eventually admits that his alcohol intake has been at least 40–50 units per week for the last 20 years. His alcohol intake has increased further during the last year after his marriage had ended.

Further investigations include the measurement of hepatitis viral serology, which was negative, and an ultrasound of the abdomen. Ultrasound showed moderate ascites, a slight reduction in liver size and an increase in splenic length of 2–3 cm. There was no evidence of a hepatoma. These findings indicate that portal hypertension has developed.

The crucial aim in management is to impress upon the patient the necessity to stop drinking alcohol and to affect this by attending an alcohol addiction unit. Acute management should include an alcohol withdrawal regimen with diazepam or chlordiazepoxide to reduce the risk of withdrawal seizures. Attention needs to be paid to nutrition. Intravenous thiamine should be given to prevent Wernicke's encephalopathy. Vitamin K is used to correct clotting abnormalities. An ascitic tap should be performed to exclude spontaneous bacterial peritonitis (which maybe asymptomatic). Treatment of ascites includes a low sodium diet and spironolactone. Daily weights should be used to measure fluid losses. Therapeutic paracentesis with concomitant albumin infusion can be used if the ascites is diuretic resistant or very uncomfortable. Surveillance endoscopy and banding of oesophageal varices should be considered in this patient, as there is evidence of portal hypertension. If oesophageal varices are present, propranolol can be used to reduce portal hypertension and prevent further variceal formation.

In this patient attendance at the addiction unit was fitful; he continued to drink heavily, and he died 3 years later as a result of a second bleed from oesophageal varices.

 KEY POINTS

- Patients who drink excessive amounts of alcohol will often disguise this fact in their history
- Alcoholic liver disease has a poor prognosis if the alcohol intake is not terminated.

CASE 8: ANOREXIA AND FEVER

History

A 22-year-old man presented with malaise and anorexia for 1 week. He vomited on one occasion, with no blood. He has felt feverish but has not taken his temperature. For 2 weeks he has had aching pains in the knees, elbows and wrists without any obvious swelling of the joints. He has not noticed any change in his urine or bowels.

Five years ago he had glandular fever confirmed serologically. He smokes 25 cigarettes per day and drinks 20–40 units of alcohol per week. He has taken marijuana and ecstasy occasionally over the past 2 years and various tablets and mixtures at clubs without being sure of the constituents. He denies any intravenous drug use. He has had irregular homosexual contacts but says that he has always used protection. He claims to have had an HIV test that was negative 6 months earlier. He has not travelled abroad in the last 2 years.

He is unemployed and lives in a flat with three other people. There is no relevant family history.

Examination

He has a temperature of 38.6°C and looks unwell. He looks as if he may be a little jaundiced. He is a little tender in the right upper quadrant of the abdomen. There are no abnormalities to find on examination of the joints or in any other system.

INVESTIGATIONS

		Normal
Haemoglobin	14.1 g/dL	13.3–17.7 g/dL
Mean corpuscular volume (MCV)	85 fL	80–99 fL
White cell count	11.5 × 10⁹/L	3.9–10.6 × 10⁹/L
Platelets	286 × 10⁹/L	150–440 × 10⁹/L
Prothrombin time	17 s	10–14 s
Sodium	135 mmol/L	135–145 mmol/L
Potassium	3.5 mmol/L	3.5–5.0 mmol/L
Urea	3.2 mmol/L	2.5–6.7 mmol/L
Creatinine	64 µmol/L	70–120 µmol/L
Bilirubin	50 mmol/L	3–17 mmol/L
Alkaline phosphatase	376 IU/L	30–300 IU/L
Alanine aminotransferase	570 IU/L	5–35 IU/L
Fasting glucose	4.1 mmol/L	4.0–6.0 mmol/L

Questions

- What is your interpretation of the findings?
- What is the likely diagnosis?
- What treatment is required?

ANSWER 8

The diagnosis is likely to be acute viral hepatitis. The biochemical results show abnormal liver function tests with a predominant change in the transaminases, indicating a hepatocellular rather than an obstructive problem in the liver. This might be caused by hepatitis A, B or C. The raised white count is compatible with acute hepatitis. Homosexuality and intravenous drug abuse are risk factors for hepatitis B and C. Other viral infections, such as cytomegalovirus and herpes simplex virus, are possible. As the drug ingestion history is unclear, there is a possibility of a drug-induced hepatitis. The prodromal joint symptoms suggest a viral infection as the cause, and this is more common with hepatitis B. Serological tests can be used to see whether there are immunoglobulin M (IgM) antibodies indicating acute infection with one of these viruses, to confirm the diagnosis. Viral loads can also be measured. The reported negative HIV test 6 months earlier makes an HIV-associated condition unlikely although patients are not always reliable in their accounts of HIV tests, and HIV seroconversion should also be considered.

This man has acute hepatitis B infection. About 30% of cases develop jaundice. Treatment is basically supportive in the acute phase. Antiviral drugs are not indicated in the vast majority of patients with acute hepatitis B. The prothrombin time in this patient is raised slightly but not enough to be an anxiety or an indicator of very severe disease. Liver function will need to be measured to monitor enzyme levels as a guide to progress. Alcohol and any other hepatotoxic drug intake should be avoided until liver function tests are back to normal. Rare complications of the acute illness are fulminant hepatic failure, aplastic anaemia, myocarditis and vasculitis. The opportunity should be taken to advise him about the potential dangers of his intake of cigarettes, drugs and alcohol, and of sexually transmitted diseases and to offer him appropriate support in these areas. HBV can survive outside the body for some time and he should advise his flatmates not to share razors and toothbrushes with him. They should consider being vaccinated. Only about 5% of adults with acute hepatitis B will develop chronic infection. Patients with alcoholic liver disease who are infected with hepatitis B have a worse liver prognosis.

 KEY POINTS

- Viral hepatitis is often associated with a prodrome of arthralgia and flu-like symptoms.
- Confirmatory evidence should be sought for patients' reports of HIV test results.
- Sexual transmission and intravenous drug use are the main methods of transmission of hepatitis B in adults in the developed world.
- Acute hepatitis B infection is a notifiable disease in the UK.

RENAL

CASE 9: TIREDNESS

History

An 85-year-old woman is investigated by her general practitioner (GP) for increasing tiredness, which has developed over the past 6 months. She has lost her appetite and feels constantly nauseated. She has lost about 8 kg in weight over the past 6 months. For the last 4 weeks she has also complained of generalized itching and cramps. She has been hypertensive for 20 years and has been on antihypertensive medication for that time. She has had two cerebrovascular accidents, which have left her with some left side weakness and reduced mobility. She is an African Caribbean, having emigrated to the United Kingdom in the 1960s. She lives alone but uses a 'meals-on-wheels' service and goes to a day hospital twice a week. She has two daughters.

Examination

Her conjunctivae are pale. Her pulse is 88/min regular, blood pressure 190/110 mmHg; mild pitting oedema of her ankles is present. Otherwise, examination of her cardiovascular and respiratory systems is normal. Neurological examination shows a left upper motor neurone facial palsy with mild weakness and increased tone and reflexes in the left arm and leg. She is able to walk with a stick. Fundoscopy shows arteriovenous nipping and increased tortuosity of the arteries.

INVESTIGATIONS

		Normal
Haemoglobin	7.8 g/dL	11.7–15.7 g/dL
Mean corpuscular volume (MCV)	84 fL	80–99 fL
White cell count	6.3×10^9/L	$3.5–11.0 \times 10^9$/L
Platelets	294×10^9/L	$150–440 \times 10^9$/L
Sodium	136 mmol/L	135–145 mmol/L
Potassium	4.8 mmol/L	3.5–5.0 mmol/L
Urea	46.2 mmol/L	2.5–6.7 mmol/L
Creatinine	769 µmol/L	70–120 µmol/L
Glucose	4.4 mmol/L	4.0–6.0 mmol/L
Albumin	37 g/L	35–50 g/L
Calcium	1.94 mmol/L	2.12–2.65 mmol/L
Phosphate	3.4 mmol/L	0.8–1.45 mmol/L
Bilirubin	15 mmol/L	3–17 mmol/L
Alanine transaminase	23 IU/L	5–35 IU/L
Alkaline phosphatase	423 IU/L	30–300 IU/L

Urinalysis: 1 protein; 1 blood
Blood film: normochromic, normocytic anaemia

Questions
- What is the diagnosis?
- How would you investigate and manage this patient?

ANSWER 9

This patient presents anorexia, nausea, weight loss, fatigue, pruritus and cramps. These are typical symptoms of end stage kidney failure.

The elevated urea and creatinine levels confirm renal failure but do not distinguish between acute and chronic renal failure. Usually, in the former, there is evidence of either a systemic illness or some other obvious precipitating cause (e.g. use of nephrotoxic drugs/prolonged episode of hypotension), whereas in the latter there is a prolonged history of general malaise. If the patient has had previous blood tests measuring serum creatinine, these will be informative about the progression of deterioration of renal function. In this patient, the anaemia and hyperparathyroidism (raised alkaline phosphatase) are features indicating chronicity of the renal failure. The normochromic, normocytic anaemia is predominantly due to erythropoietin deficiency (the kidney is the major source of erythropoietin production). Hyperparathyroidism is a result of elevated serum phosphate levels due to decreased renal clearance of phosphate and reduced vitamin D levels (the kidney is the site of hydroxylation of 25-hydroxycholecalciferol to the active form 1,25-dihydroxycholecalciferol). A hand X-ray showing the typical appearances of hyperparathyroidism (erosion of the terminal phalanges and subperiosteal erosions of the radial aspects of the middle phalanges) can help to confirm long-standing renal failure.

Renal ultrasound is the essential investigation. Ultrasound will accurately size the kidneys and identify obvious causes for renal failure, such as polycystic kidney disease or obstruction causing bilateral hydronephrosis. Asymmetrically sized kidneys suggest reflux nephropathy or renovascular disease. In this case, ultrasound showed two small (8 cm) echogenic kidneys consistent with long-standing renal failure. A renal biopsy in this case is not appropriate as biopsies of small kidneys have a high incidence of bleeding complications, and the sample obtained would show extensive glomerular and tubulointerstitial fibrosis and may not identify the original disease. The patient's renal failure may have been due to hypertension or a primary glomerulonephritis such as immunoglobulin A (IgA) nephropathy. African-Caribbeans are more prone to develop hypertensive renal failure than other racial groups.

Antihypertensive medications are needed to treat her blood pressure adequately, oral phosphate binders and vitamin D preparations to control her secondary hyperparathyroidism, and erythropoietin injections to treat her anaemia. The case raises the dilemma of whether dialysis is appropriate in this patient. Hospital-based haemodialysis and home-based peritoneal dialysis are the options available. Her age and comorbid illnesses preclude renal transplantation. Conservative management without dialysis may be appropriate in this case.

 KEY POINTS

- Patients often become symptomatic due to renal failure only when their glomerular filtration rate (GFR) is less than 15 mL/min and thus may present with end-stage renal failure.
- Previous measurements of serum creatinine enable the rate of deterioration of renal function to be known.
- Renal ultrasound is the key imaging investigation.

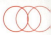

CASE 10: BACK PAIN

History

A 27-year-old woman is admitted to the emergency department complaining of pain across her back. She became unwell 2 days previously when she started to develop a fever and an ache in her back. The pain has become progressively more severe. She has vomited twice in the past 6 h. She has had no previous significant medical history apart from an uncomplicated episode of cystitis 3 months ago.

Examination

She looks unwell and is flushed. Her temperature is 39.5°C. Her pulse is 120 beats/min, and blood pressure is 104/68 mmHg. Examination of the cardiovascular and respiratory systems is unremarkable. Her abdomen is generally tender, but most markedly in both loins. Bowel sounds are normal.

🔍 INVESTIGATIONS

		Normal
Haemoglobin	15.3 g/dL	11.7–15.7 g/dL
White cell count	25.2 × 10⁹/L	3.5–11.0 × 10⁹/L
Platelets	406 × 10⁹/L	150–440 × 10⁹/L
Sodium	134 mmol/L	135–145 mmol/L
Potassium	4.1 mmol/L	3.5–5.0 mmol/L
Urea	14.2 mmol/L	2.5–6.7 mmol/L
Creatinine	106 µmol/L	70–120 µmol/L
Albumin	44 g/L	35–50 g/L
C-reactive protein (CRP)	316 mg/L	<5 mg/L

Urinalysis: ++ protein; +++ blood; ++ nitrites
Urine microscopy: >50 red cells; >50 white cells
Abdominal X-ray: normal

Questions
- What is the likely diagnosis?
- How would you investigate and manage this patient?

ANSWER 10

This woman has the symptoms and signs of acute pyelonephritis. Acute pyelonephritis is much more common in women than men and occurs due to ascent of bacteria up the urinary tract. Pregnancy, diabetes mellitus, immunosuppression and structurally abnormal urinary tracts increase the likelihood of ascending infection.

> **! Differential diagnosis**
>
> Pyelonephritis causes loin pain, which can be unilateral or bilateral. The differential diagnoses of loin pain include obstructive uropathy, renal infarction, renal cell carcinoma, renal papillary necrosis, renal calculi, glomerulonephritis, polycystic kidney disease, medullary sponge kidney and loin-pain haematuria syndrome.

Fever may be as high as 40°C with associated systemic symptoms of anorexia, nausea and vomiting. Some patients may have preceding symptoms of cystitis (dysuria, urinary frequency, urgency and haematuria), but these lower urinary tract symptoms do not always occur in patients with acute pyelonephritis. Many patients will give a history of cystitis within the previous 6 months. Elderly patients with pyelonephritis may present with nonspecific symptoms and confusion. Pyelonephritis may also mimic other conditions, such as acute appendicitis, acute cholecystitis, acute pancreatitis and lower lobe pneumonia. There is usually marked tenderness over the kidneys both posteriorly and anteriorly. Severe untreated infection may lead to septic shock.

The raised white cell count and CRP are consistent with an acute bacterial infection. Microscopic haematuria, proteinuria and leucocytes in the urine occur because of inflammation in the urinary tract. The presence of bacteria in the urine is confirmed by the reduction of nitrates to nitrites.

This woman should be admitted. Blood and urine cultures should be taken, and she should be commenced on intravenous fluids and antibiotics until the organism is identified, and then an oral antibiotic to which the organism is sensitive can be used. Initial therapy could be with gentamicin and ampicillin or ciprofloxacin. She should have a renal ultrasound scan to exclude any evidence of obstruction. In patients with obstructive uropathy, infection may lead to a pyonephrosis with severe loin pain, fever, septic shock and renal failure. If there is evidence of a hydronephrosis in the context of urinary sepsis, a nephrostomy should be inserted urgently to prevent these complications.

Patients with an uncomplicated renal infection should be treated with a 2-week course of antibiotics and then have a repeat urine culture 10–14 days after treatment has finished to confirm eradication of infection. In patients with infection complicated by stones or renal scarring, a 6-week course of treatment should be given.

 KEY POINTS

- Acute pyelonephritis may present with or without preceding lower urinary tract symptoms.
- Renal ultrasound should be performed within 24h of admission to exclude urinary tract obstruction.
- Antibiotics should be continued for at least 2 weeks in cases of acute pyelonephritis to minimize the risk of relapse.

ENDOCRINOLOGY

CASE 11: WEIGHT GAIN

History

A 64-year-old man goes to his general practitioner (GP) because he has become increasingly overweight. He has gained 8 kg in weight over the past 6 months. He has noticed that he is constantly hungry. He has found that he is bruising easily. He finds it difficult to get up from his armchair or to climb stairs. He feels depressed and finds himself waking early in the mornings. He has had no previous physical or psychiatric illnesses. He is a retired miner and lives with his wife in a terraced house. He smokes 30 cigarettes per day and drinks 15 units of alcohol per week.

Examination

He is overweight, particularly in the abdominal region. There are purple stretch marks on his abdomen and thighs. His skin is thin, and there are spontaneous bruises. His pulse is 76/min, regular, and blood pressure is 168/104 mmHg. There is peripheral oedema. Otherwise, examination of his heart, respiratory and abdominal systems is normal. His neurological examination is otherwise normal, apart from some weakness in shoulder abduction and hip flexion.

INVESTIGATIONS		
		Normal
Haemoglobin	13.2 g/dL	13.3–17.7 g/dL
Mean corpuscular volume (MCV)	87 fL	80–99 fL
White cell count	5.2 × 10⁹/L	3.9–10.6 × 10⁹/L
Platelets	237 × 10⁹/L	150–440 × 10⁹/L
Sodium	138 mmol/L	135–145 mmol/L
Potassium	3.3 mmol/L	3.5–5.0 mmol/L
Urea	6.2 mmol/L	2.5–6.7 mmol/L
Creatinine	113 µmol/L	70–120 µmol/L
Albumin	38 g/L	35–50 g/L
Glucose	8.3 mmol/L	4.0–6.0 mmol/L
Bilirubin	16 mmol/L	3–17 mmol/L
Alanine transaminase	24 IU/L	5–35 IU/L
Alkaline phosphatase	92 IU/L	30–300 IU/L
Gamma-glutamyl transpeptidase	43 IU/L	11–51 IU/L

Urinalysis: – protein; – blood; ++ glucose
Chest X-ray: normal

Questions

- What is the likely diagnosis?
- How would you investigate and manage this patient?

ANSWER 11

The symptoms and signs of proximal myopathy, striae and truncal obesity are features of Cushing's syndrome. Fat accumulation causes a "moon face", a "buffalo hump" and enlarged fat pads in the supraclavicular fossae. The hyperglycaemia and hypokalaemia would fit this diagnosis. In addition psychiatric disturbances, typically depression, may occur in Cushing's syndrome. Cushing's disease is due to a pituitary adenoma secreting adrenocorticotrophic hormone (ACTH). The term *Cushing's syndrome* is a wider one and encompasses a group of disorders caused by overproduction of cortisol.

! **Causes of Cushing's syndrome**

- ACTH secretion by a basophil adenoma of the anterior pituitary gland (Cushing's disease).
- Ectopic ACTH secretion (e.g. from a bronchial carcinoma), often causing a massive release of cortisol and a severe and rapid onset of symptoms.
- Primary adenoma/carcinoma of the adrenal cortex (suppressed ACTH).
- Iatrogenic: corticosteroid treatment. This is the commonest cause in day-to-day clinical practice.

This patient's primary presenting complaint is rapid-onset obesity. The principal causes of obesity are

- genetic;
- environmental: excessive food intake, lack of exercise;
- hormonal: hypothyroidism, Cushing's syndrome, polycystic ovaries and hyperprolactinaemia; and
- alcohol-induced pseudo-Cushing's syndrome.

This patient should be investigated by an endocrinologist. The first point is to establish that this man has abnormal cortisol secretion. There should be loss of the normal diurnal rhythm with an elevated midnight cortisol level or increased urinary conjugated cortisol excretion. A dexamethasone suppression test would normally suppress cortisol excretion. It is then important to exclude common causes of abnormal cortisol excretion, such as stress/depression or alcohol abuse. Measurement of ACTH levels distinguishes between adrenal (low ACTH) and pituitary/ectopic (high ACTH) causes. This patient drinks alcohol moderately and has a normal gamma-glutamyl transpeptidase. His depression seems to be a consequence of his cortisol excess rather than a cause as he has no psychiatric history.

His ACTH level is elevated. Bronchial carcinoma is a possibility as he is a heavy smoker, and the onset of his Cushing's syndrome has been rapid. However his chest X-ray is normal. In this man a magnetic resonance imaging (MRI) scan (T1-weighted coronal image) through the pituitary shows a hypointense microadenoma (Figure 11.1, arrow). This can be treated with surgery or radiotherapy. Transsphenoidal microadenomectomy is the treatment of choice as it cures the patient and leaves them with normal hypothalamic–pituitary–adrenal function.

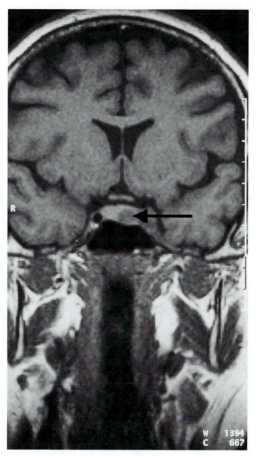

Figure 11.1 Magnetic resonance imaging scan through the pituitary.

 KEY POINTS

- Patients with rapid-onset obesity should have endocrine causes excluded.
- Corticosteroid treatment is the commonest cause for Cushing's syndrome.
- Patients with severe and rapid-onset Cushing's syndrome often have ectopic ACTH secretion or cortisol-secreting adrenal tumours.

CASE 12: PERSONALITY CHANGE

History
A 62-year-old woman is encouraged to consult her general practitioner because her husband thinks she has become rather confused and irritable over the last 3–4 weeks. She admits to feeling rather irritable and has found it difficult to remember lists on occasions. There is no relevant medical history.

On systems review she complains of some non-specific back pain. This has been present for 2 months and is maximal in the low thoracic area. She does not recall any trauma at the start of the problem and the pain is gradually increasing in severity. It is partially relieved by paracetamol and ibuprofen that she buys in the local pharmacy. She has noticed some abdominal discomfort and constipation which she has related to the medication for the back pain. She takes no other medicines and does not drink or smoke.

Examination
She looks a little pale. There is no abdominal tenderness. Bowel sounds are normal. She has tenderness locally over the lower thoracic spine.

INVESTIGATIONS

		Normal
Haemoglobin	9.9 g/dL	11.7–15.7 g/dL
White cell count	3.2×10^9/L	$3.5–11.0 \times 10^9$/L
Platelets	112×10^9/L	$150–440 \times 10^9$/L
Sodium	140 mmol/L	135–145 mmol/L
Erythrocyte sedimentation rate (ESR)	96 mm/hr	<10 mm/hr
Potassium	3.8 mmol/L	3.5–5.0 mmol/L
Urea	7.5 mmol/L	2.5–6.7 mmol/L
Creatinine	131 µmol/L	70–120 µmol/L
Random glucose	5.1 mmol/L	4.0–6.0 mmol/L

Questions
- What is the most likely diagnosis?
- What other investigations would you perform?

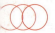

ANSWER 12

There are a number of clues here that there is a significant problem. She presents with a combination of character change, back pain, abdominal pain and constipation. Abdominal pain and constipation might be related to opiate analgesic therapy but not to paracetamol and ibuprofen. The abnormal findings of low values for haemoglobin, white cells and platelets and mildly abnormal renal function are found in the investigations.

The haematological investigations suggest that there is a bone marrow problem which is likely to be related to the bony tenderness in the thoracic spine. The character change and the abdominal symptoms, with the finding of a possible bony problem, raise the possibility of hypercalcaemia which would explain all these findings.

The clinical manifestations of hypercalcaemia include confusion, reduced concentration, fatigue, muscle weakness, abdominal pain, nausea, constipation, polydipsia, polyuria, dehydration, nephrolithiasis, hypertension, short QT on ECG, bone changes (osteitis fibrosa cystica, brown tumours).

90% of cases of hypercalcaemia are related to primary hyperparathyroidism or malignancy, with multiple myeloma as a common malignancy. Other causes are

> **!**
>
> - sarcoidosis
> - ectopic hormone production in squamous cell lung cancer
> - tertiary hyperparathyroidism (in renal failure)
> - thyrotoxicosis
> - vitamin D intoxication
> - thiazide diuretics (mild hypercalcaemia)
> - adrenal insufficiency
> - tuberculosis

The investigations indicating bone marrow depression here and the bone pain suggest that malignancy is the likely cause. The high ESR could be compatible with any disseminated malignancy but is characteristic of multiple myeloma.

The important first investigations here are to confirm the hypercalcaemia and to investigate the back pain. When interpreting serum calcium the serum albumin should be measured and the calcium level corrected for abnormalities in albumin. Also the serum phosphate may help, being usually low in hyperparathyroidism and high in malignancy. In the presence of hypercalcaemia the parathyroid hormone level will be below normal unless there is hyperparathyroidism.

In this case the serum calcium and phosphate were both raised and the X-rays of the thoracic spine and skull (see Figure 12.1) showed lytic bone lesions typical of multiple myeloma. Plain X-rays are preferred to a radio-isotope bone scan which may not show hot spots from radio-isotope accumulation in osteoblasts typical of other malignant bone involvement.

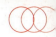

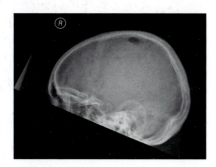

Figure 12.1 Skull X-ray

The diagnosis was confirmed with protein electrophoresis which showed a monoclonal band in the gamma region and by bone marrow biopsy showing an accumulation of abnormal plasma cells. Myeloma occurs in around 1–4/100,000 adults per year and is treated by steroids and chemotherapy and by stem cell transplants. Remissions are common but cure is unusual.

 KEY POINTS

- Hypercalcaemia symptoms are traditionally stones, bones, abdominal groans and psyche moans but symptoms may be non-specific.
- Back pain requires investigation when associated with other features such as neurological symptoms or investigations suggesting malignancy or infection.

NEUROLOGY

CASE 13: A WEAK HAND

History

A 67-year-old man is referred to a neurologist by his general practitioner (GP). His symptoms are of weakness and wasting of the muscles of his left hand. He has noticed the weakness is worse after using his hand, for example, after using a screwdriver. He has also noticed cramps in his forearm muscles. On a few occasions recently he has felt choking sensations after taking fluids. Past medical history is notable for hypertension for 15 years and a myocardial infarction 3 years previously. Medication consists of simvastatin, aspirin and atenolol. He is a retired university lecturer. He lives with his wife, and they have two grown-up children. He is a non-smoker and drinks a bottle of wine a week.

Examination

Blood pressure is 146/88 mmHg. There are no abnormalities in the cardiovascular or respiratory systems or the abdomen. There is some wasting of the muscles in the upper limbs, particularly in the left hand. There is some fasciculation in the muscles of the forearms bilaterally. Power is globally reduced in the left hand and slightly reduced in the right hand. Muscle tone is normal. The biceps and triceps jerks are brisk bilaterally. There is no sensory loss. There is slight dysarthria.

Questions

- What is the diagnosis?
- What is the prognosis?

ANSWER 13

This man has evidence of lower motor neurone problems in the hands with weakness, wasting and fasciculation. The most likely diagnosis is motor neurone disease. This is a degenerative disease of unknown cause that affects the motor neurones of the spinal cord, the cranial nerve nuclei, and the motor cortex. The disease usually presents between the ages of 50 and 70 years.

Weakness and wasting of the muscles of one hand or arm is the commonest presentation. Weakness is most marked after exertion. Painful cramps of the forearm muscles are common in the early phases of the disease. Patients may present with lower limb weakness or with dysarthria or dysphagia. The characteristic physical sign of this condition is fasciculation, which is an irregular rapid contraction of segments of muscle, caused by denervation of the muscle from a lower motor neurone lesion. As in this man, reflexes can be brisk due to loss of cortical motor neurones. There is no sensory loss.

Motor neurone disease is divided into five types:

- amyotrophic lateral sclerosis (commonest, upper and lower motor neurone)
- primary lateral sclerosis (upper motor neurone)
- progressive muscular atrophy (lower motor neurone)
- progressive bulbar palsy (bulbar lower motor neurone)
- pseudobulbar palsy (bulbar upper motor neurone)

In advanced cases diagnosis is easy, but early cases are more problematic. Limb weakness worsening with fatigue may be confused with myasthenia gravis. Dysphagia and dysarthria in the elderly are much more commonly due to the pseudobulbar palsy of cerebrovascular disease. Cervical myelopathy is another common cause of wasting and fasciculation of the upper limbs without sensory loss. Brachial plexus lesions from trauma or invasion by an apical lung tumour (Pancoast tumour) may affect one arm. A predominant motor peripheral neuropathy causes a symmetrical pattern of weakness, and reflexes are reduced.

Unfortunately motor neurone disease is a progressive and incurable condition. Patients tend to develop a spastic weakness of the legs. Bulbar palsy causes dysarthria and dysphasia. Sphincter function is usually not affected. Intellect is generally not affected.

There is no curative treatment for this condition. The mean duration of survival from presentation is between 2 and 4 years. The patient and his family will have to be told of the diagnosis and prognosis. Support must be given by a multidisciplinary team. As the disease progresses and speech deteriorates communication may be helped by computer-linked devices. A feeding gastrostomy may be required to enable adequate calorie intake. Non-invasive ventilation can be used to help respiratory failure, but death usually occurs from bronchopneumonia.

 KEY POINTS

- Motor neuron disease most commonly starts with weakness and wasting of the muscles of one hand.
- Fasciculation of the muscles is characteristic of this condition.
- The absence of sensory loss helps in the differential diagnosis.

CASE 14: DOUBLE VISION

History

A 43-year-old woman presents to her general practitioner (GP) complaining of diplopia, more marked in the evenings, for the last 3 months. She has noticed difficulty holding her head up, again especially in the evenings. She has problems finishing a meal because of difficulty chewing. Her husband and friends have noticed that her voice has become quieter. She has lost about 3 kg in weight in the past 6 months. The woman has had no significant previous medical illnesses. She lives with her husband and three children. She is a non-smoker and drinks about 15 units of alcohol per week. She is taking no regular medication.

Examination

She looks well, and examination of the cardiovascular, respiratory and abdominal systems is normal. Power in all muscle groups is grossly normal but seems to decrease after testing a movement repetitively. Tone, coordination, reflexes and sensation are normal. Bilateral ptosis is present and is exacerbated by prolonged upward gaze. Pupillary reflexes, eye movements and fundoscopy are normal.

Questions

- What is the diagnosis?
- What are the major differential diagnoses?
- How would you investigate and manage this patient?

ANSWER 14

This woman's generalized weakness is caused by myasthenia gravis. Myasthenia gravis is due to the presence of acetylcholine receptor antibodies causing impaired neuromuscular transmission. It characteristically affects the external ocular, bulbar, neck and shoulder girdle muscles. Weakness is worse after repetitive movements, which cause acetylcholine depletion from the presynaptic terminals. The onset is usually gradual. Ptosis of the upper lids is often associated with diplopia due to weakness of the external ocular muscles. Speech may become soft when the patient is tired. Symptoms are usually worse in the evenings and better in the mornings. Permanent paralysis eventually develops in some muscle groups. In severe cases respiratory weakness occurs.

> **❗ Differential diagnoses of generalized muscle weakness**
>
> - *Motor neurone disease*: suggested clinically by muscle fasciculation and later by marked muscle weakness.
> - *Muscular dystrophies*: selective muscular weakness occurs in specific diseases (e.g. facioscapulohumeral dystrophy). There is usually a family history.
> - *Dystrophia myotonica*: this causes ptosis, wasting of the masseter, temporal and sternomastoid muscles and distal muscular atrophy. There is a characteristic facial appearance with frontal baldness, expressionless facies and sunken cheeks. There may be gonadal atrophy and mental retardation. There is usually a family history. The electromyogram (EMG) is diagnostic.
> - *Polymyositis*: this may have an acute or chronic onset. A skin rash and joint pains are common. The creatine kinase level is raised, and a muscle biopsy is diagnostic.
> - *Miscellaneous myopathies*: thyrotoxic, hypothyroid, Cushing's, alcoholic.
> - *Non-metastatic associations of malignancy*: thymoma is associated with myasthenia gravis in 10 per cent of cases; the Eaton–Lambert myasthenic syndrome is associated with small-cell lung carcinoma.

This patient should be investigated by a neurologist. The EMG will demonstrate fatiguability in response to repetitive supramaximal stimulation. Intravenous injection of edrophonium (Tensilon) will increase muscular power for a few minutes. Blood should be assayed for acetylcholine receptor antibodies (present in 90 per cent). Computed tomography (CT) of the thorax should be performed to detect the presence of a thymoma or lung cancer. Corticosteroids are the drugs of first choice. Anticholinesterase drugs greatly improve muscle power but have many side effects. Thymectomy should be considered. It is most effective within 5 years of diagnosis and when there is no thymoma.

> **🔑 KEY POINTS**
>
> - Myasthenia gravis is a cause of abnormal muscular fatiguability.
> - In its initial stages it affects certain characteristic muscle groups.

RHEUMATOLOGY

CASE 15: PAINFUL KNEE

History

A 35-year-old man is seen in the emergency department because he has developed a painful, swollen right knee. This has occurred rapidly over the past 36 h. There is no history of trauma to the knee or previous joint problems. He feels generally unwell and has also noticed his eyes are sore. He has had no significant previous medical illnesses. He is married with two children. He is a non-smoker and drinks about 15 units of alcohol per week. He is a businessman and returned 3 weeks ago from a business trip to Thailand.

Examination

His temperature is 38.0°C. Both eyes appear red. There is a brown macular rash on his palms and soles. Examination of cardiovascular, respiratory, abdominal and neurological systems is normal. His right knee is swollen, hot and tender with limitation in flexion. No other joint appears to be affected.

INVESTIGATIONS		
		Normal
Haemoglobin	13.8 g/dL	13.3–17.7 g/dL
Mean corpuscular volume (MCV)	87 fL	80–99 fL
White cell count	13.6 × 10⁹/L	3.9–10.6 × 10⁹/L
Platelets	345 × 10⁹/L	150–440 × 10⁹/L
Erythrocyte sedimentation rate (ESR)	64 mm/h	<10 mm/h
Sodium	139 mmol/L	135–145 mmol/L
Potassium	4.1 mmol/L	3.5–5.0 mmol/L
Urea	5.2 mmol/L	2.5–6.7 mmol/L
Creatinine	94 µmol/L	70–120 µmol/L

Urinalysis: no protein; no blood; no glucose
Blood cultures: negative
X-ray of the knee: soft-tissue swelling around joint

Questions
- What is the diagnosis and what are the major differential diagnoses?
- How would you investigate and manage this patient?

ANSWER 15

This patient has a monoarthropathy, a rash and red eyes. Investigations show a raised white cell count and ESR. The diagnosis in this man was postinfective inflammatory mucositis and arthritis, often shortened to reactive arthritis, and also known as Reiter's syndrome. This disease classically presents with a triad of symptoms (although all three may not always be present):

- seronegative arthritis affecting mainly lower limb joints
- conjunctivitis
- non-specific urethritis (NSU).

The trigger can be non-gonococcal urethritis (*Chlamydia trachomatis*)) or certain enteric infections (*Salmonella, Shigella, Yerinia* and *Campylobacter*. This patient is likely to have contracted NSU after sexual intercourse in Thailand. On direct questioning he admitted to the presence of a urethral discharge. The acute arthritis is typically a monoarthritis but can develop into a chronic relapsing destructive arthritis affecting the knees and feet and causing sacroiliitis and spondylitis. Tendinitis and plantar fasciitis may occur. The red eyes are due to conjunctivitis and anterior uveitis and can recur with flares of the arthritis. The rash on the patient's palmar surfaces is the characteristic brown macular rash of this condition: kerato-dermablenorrhagica. Other features of this condition that are sometimes seen include nail dystrophy and a circinate balanitis. Systemic manifestations such as pericarditis, pleuritis, fever and lymphadenopathy may occur in this disease. The ESR is usually elevated.

> **! Differential diagnoses of an acute monoarthritis**
>
> - *Gonococcal arthritis*: occasionally a polyarthritis affecting the small joints of the hands and wrists, with a pustular rash.
> - *Acute septic arthritis*: the patient looks ill and septic, and the skin over the joint is very erythematous.
> - *Other seronegative arthritides*: ankylosing spondylitis, psoriatic arthropathy.
> - *Viral arthritis*: usually polyarticular.
> - *Acute rheumatoid arthritis*: usually polyarticular.
> - *Acute gout*: most commonly affects the metatarsophalangeal joints.
> - *Pseudogout*: caused by sodium pyrophosphate crystals; often affects large joints in older patients.
> - *Lyme disease*: caused by *Borrelia burgdorfii* infection transmitted by a tick bite; may have the characteristic skin rash: erythema chronicum migrans.
> - *Haemorrhagic arthritis*: usually a history of trauma or bleeding disorder.

This patient should have urethral swabs taken to exclude chlamydial/gonococcal infections and the appropriate antibiotics given. His knee should be aspirated. A Gram stain will exclude a pyogenic infection, and birefringent microscopy can be used to detect uric acid or pyrophosphate crystals. This patient should be given non-steroidal anti-inflammatory drugs (NSAIDs) for the pain, and he may require intraarticular steroids or oral prednisolone. Sulfasalazine is used in refractory cases.. If his disease relapses he should be referred to a rheumatologist. He and his wife should be referred to the sexually transmitted disease clinic for counselling and testing for other sexually transmitted diseases, such as hepatitis B, HIV and syphilis.

> **KEY POINTS**
>
> - The most likely causes of an acute large joint monoarthritis are a septic arthritis and a seronegative arthritis.
> - Septic arthritis must be recognized and treated as a medical emergency as it can cause rapid destruction of the joint and septicaemia.

CASE 16: PAIN IN THE KNEE

History
An 80-year-old woman presents to her general practitioner (GP) with pain and swelling in her left knee. The pain began 2 days previously, and she says that the knee is now hot, swollen and painful on movement. In the past she has a history of mild osteoarthritis of the hips. She has occasional heartburn and indigestion. She had a health check 6 months previously and was told that everything was fine except for some elevation of her blood pressure, which was 172/102 mmHg, and her creatinine level, which was around the upper limit of normal. The blood pressure was checked several times over the next 4 weeks and found to be persistently elevated, and she was started on treatment with 2.5 mg bendroflumethiazide. The last blood pressure reading was 148/84 mmHg. There is no relevant family history. She has never smoked, and her alcohol consumption averages four units per week. She takes occasional paracetamol for hip pain.

Examination
Her blood pressure is 142/86 mmHg. The temperature is 37.5°C, and the pulse is 88/min. There is grade 2 hypertensive retinopathy. There is no other abnormality on cardiovascular or respiratory examination. In the hands there are Heberden's nodes over the distal interphalangeal joints.

The left knee is hot and swollen with evidence of effusion in the joint with a positive patellar tap. There is pain on flexion beyond 90 degrees. The right knee appears normal.

🔍 INVESTIGATIONS		
		Normal
Haemoglobin	12.1 g/dL	11.7–15.7 g/dL
White cell count	12.4 × 10⁹/L	3.5–11.0 × 10⁹/L
Platelets	384 × 10⁹/L	150–440 × 10⁹/L
Erythrocyte sedimentation rate (ESR)	48 mm/h	<10 mm/h
Sodium	136 mmol/L	135–145 mmol/L
Potassium	3.6 mmol/L	3.5–5.0 mmol/L
Urea	7.3 mmol/L	2.5–6.7 mmol/L
Creatinine	116 µmol/L	70–120 µmol/L
Glucose	10.8 mmol/L	4.0–6.0 mmol/L

An X-ray of the knees is performed, and the result is shown in Figure 16.1.

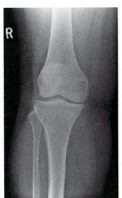 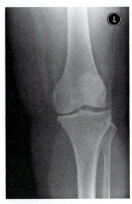

Questions
- What is the likely diagnosis?
- What is the appropriate management?

Figure 16.1 X-ray of both knees.

ANSWER 16

The clinical picture is one of an acute monoarthritis. The patient has a history of some hip pains, but this and the Heberden's nodes are common findings in an 80-year-old woman, related to osteoarthritis. The blood results show a raised white cell count and ESR, a raised blood sugar, and renal function at the upper limit of normal.

> **! Differential diagnoses of pain in the knee**
>
> The differential diagnosis includes trauma, septic arthritis, gout and pseudogout.

The recent introduction of a thiazide diuretic for treatment of the hypertension increases the suspicion of gout. Pseudogout is caused by deposition of calcium pyrophosphate crystals and would be expected to show calcification in the articular cartilage in the knee joint. The X-rays here show some joint space narrowing but no evidence of calcification in the articular cartilage. The fever, high white cell count and ESR are compatible with acute gout. The raised glucose may also be a side effect of thiazide diuretics. If this remains after the acute arthritis has subsided, then it may need further treatment. Precipitation of gout by thiazides is more likely in older women, particularly in the presence of renal impairment and diabetes. It may involve the hands, be polyarticular, and can affect existing Heberden's nodes.

The serum uric acid level is likely to be raised, but this occurs commonly without evidence of acute gout. The definitive investigation is aspiration of the joint. The fluid should be sent for culture and inspection with a specific request for inspection for crystals. A high white cell count would be expected in an acute inflammatory arthritis. The diagnosis is made from the needle-like crystals of uric acid, which are negatively birefringent under polarized light, unlike the positively birefringent crystals of calcium pyrophosphate.

In this case the pain in the joint was partly relieved by the aspiration. Treatment with a non-steroidal anti-inflammatory drug should be covered by a proton pump inhibitor in view of her history of heartburn and indigestion. The thiazide diuretic was changed to an angiotensin-converting enzyme inhibitor as treatment for her hypertension, and the blood glucose elevation resolved. A short course of prednisolone can also be used in acute gout. A xanthine oxidase inhibitor such as allopurinol might be considered if the serum urate remained raised or the condition did not settle after stopping the thiazide diuretic.

> **⚷ KEY POINTS**
>
> - A careful drug history is an essential part of the history.
> - Thiazide diuretics can precipitate diabetes and gout, especially in the elderly.

HAEMATOLOGY

CASE 17: EASY BRUISING

History

A 68-year-old woman presents to her general practitioner (GP) complaining of spontaneous bruising mainly on her legs. The bruising has been noticeable over the last 3 weeks. She cannot remember any episodes of trauma. She has suffered a major nosebleed. She feels very tired and has noticed shortness of breath on exertion. There is no significant past medical history. There is no family history of a bleeding disorder. She is a non-smoker and drinks a small amount of alcohol socially.

Examination

On examination there are multiple areas of purpura on her legs and to a lesser extent on her abdomen and arms. The purpuric lesions vary in colour from black–purple to yellow. She is pale with conjunctival pallor. There are two bullae in the mouth, and there is spontaneous bleeding from the gums. There are multiple small retinal haemorrhages on fundoscopy. Blood pressure is 118/72 mmHg. Examination of the cardiovascular, respiratory and abdominal systems is unremarkable.

INVESTIGATIONS		
		Normal
Haemoglobin	5.8 g/dL	11.7–15.7 g/dL
Mean corpuscular volume (MCV)	83 fL	80–99 fL
White cell count	14.1×10^9/L	$3.5–11.0 \times 10^9$/L
Platelets	9×10^9/L	$150–440 \times 10^9$/L
Sodium	139 mmol/L	135–145 mmol/L
Potassium	4.6 mmol/L	3.5–5.0 mmol/L
Urea	4.4 mmol/L	2.5–6.7 mmol/L
Creatinine	85 µmol/L	70–120 µmol/L
Glucose	4.3 mmol/L	4.0–6.0 mmol/L

Clotting screen: normal

Questions
- What is the differential diagnosis?
- How would you further investigate and manage this patient?

ANSWER 17

The combination of anaemia, neutropenia and thrombocytopenia is termed pancytopenia. Causes of severe pancytopenia include aplastic anaemia, vitamin B_{12} or folate deficiency, haematological malignancy such as myelodysplasia or leukaemia and tuberculosis.

This woman has spontaneous bruising due to acute myeloid leukaemia (AML). She has profound thrombocytopenia with a platelet count of 9×10^9/L. An increased tendency to bleed or bruise can be due to platelet, coagulation or blood vessel abnormalities. Platelet/vessel wall defects cause spontaneous purpura in the skin and mucous membranes or immediately after trauma. A lack of a history of trauma and frequent severe bruising raises the possibility of a bleeding diathesis. Disorders of platelet function usually cause immediate bleeding after a procedure whereas coagulation defects cause haematomas and haemarthroses usually with a time delay after trauma. The age of onset of bleeding may distinguish between a congenital and an acquired cause of bleeding. The onset of bleeding in later life suggests an acquired condition. Family history may identify a condition such as haemophilia. The distribution of bruising may also suggest the diagnosis. Thrombocytopenic purpura is most evident over the ankles and pressure areas. Retinal haemorrhages tend to occur if there is a combination of severe thrombocytopenia and anaemia. Senile purpura and steroid-induced bruising occur mainly on the forearms and backs of the hands. Henoch–Schönlein purpura typically occurs over the extensor aspects of the limbs and buttocks. Scurvy causes bleeding from the gums and around the hair follicles. Non-accidental injury in children can present with bruising. It is important to take a dietary and drug history. Drugs which can cause bruising include anticoagulants, antiplatelet drugs and steroids.

Petechiae are small capillary haemorrhages that characteristically develop in crops in areas of increased venous pressure, such as the dependent parts of the body. Petechiae are the smallest bleeding lesions (pinhead in size), and suggest problems with platelet number or function. Purpura are larger in size than petechiae with variable shape and involve bleeding into subcutaneous tissues. Purpura can be seen in a variety of bleeding disorders, including thrombocytopenia and coagulation cascade disorders. Palpable purpura can be seen in vasculitic processes such as Henoch–Schönlein purpura.

AML is the most common acute leukaemia in adults with a mean age at presentation of 65 years. Patients with AML generally present with symptoms related to complications of pancytopenia (eg, anemia, neutropenia, and thrombocytopenia), including weakness, breathlessness and easy fatigability, infections of variable severity, and/or haemorrhagic findings such as gingival bleeding, ecchymoses, epistaxis, or menorrhagia. Most patients will have blasts on the peripheral blood smear and the diagnosis is confirmed by the results of a bone marrow examination. Blast forms must account for at least 20% of the total cellularity of the bone marrow sample.

This patient should be immediately referred to a haematology unit. Platelet transfusion is usually given if there is significant bleeding or the platelet count is less than 15×10^9/L to prevent a major spontaneous bleed. Initial investigations are examination of the peripheral blood smear and performing a bone marrow aspirate.

KEY POINTS

- A careful history and examination can help in the diagnosis of easy bruising. The patient should be asked about associated trauma, location and severity of bruising, bleeding history with previous procedures, nutrition, medication use, and family history.

- The differential diagnosis of pancytopenia with peripheral blasts includes AML, myelodysplasia, a blast crisis from a chronic myeloid leukaemia, a mixed phenotype acute leukaemia, folate or B12 deficiency and miliary tuberculosis.

CASE 18: TIREDNESS, BREATHLESSNESS AND HEADACHES

History

A 63-year-old woman goes to her general practitioner (GP) complaining of extreme tiredness. She has been increasingly fatigued over the past year, but in recent weeks she has become breathless on exertion and light-headed and complained of headaches. Her feet have become numb, and she has started to become unsteady on her feet. She has had no significant previous medical illnesses. She is a retired teacher and lives alone. Until the last 2 years she was active, walking 3 or 4 miles a day. She is a non-smoker and drinks about 15 units of alcohol per week. She is taking no regular medication. Her mother and one of her two sisters have thyroid problems.

Examination

Her conjunctivae are pale, and sclerae are yellow. Her temperature is 37.8°C. Her pulse rate is 96/min and regular, and blood pressure is 142/72 mmHg. Examination of her cardiovascular, respiratory and abdominal systems is normal. She has a symmetrical distal weakness affecting her arms and legs. Knee and ankle jerks are absent, and she has extensor plantar responses. She has sensory loss in a glove-and-stocking distribution with a particularly severe loss of joint position sense.

INVESTIGATIONS

		Normal
Haemoglobin	4.2 g/dL	11.7–15.7 g/dL
Mean corpuscular volume (MCV)	112 fL	80–99 fL
White cell count	3.3×10^9/L	$3.5–11.0 \times 10^9$/L
Platelets	102×10^9/L	$150–440 \times 10^9$/L
Sodium	136 mmol/L	135–145 mmol/L
Potassium	4.4 mmol/L	3.5–5.0 mmol/L
Urea	5.2 mmol/L	2.5–6.7 mmol/L
Creatinine	92 µmol/L	70–120 µmol/L
Glucose	4.4 mmol/L	4.0–6.0 mmol/L
Bilirubin	45 mmol/L	3–17 mmol/L
Alanine transaminase	33 IU/L	5–35 IU/L
Alkaline phosphatase	263 IU/L	30–300 IU/L

Questions

- What is the diagnosis?
- How would you investigate and manage this patient?

ANSWER 18

This patient has a severe macrocytic anaemia and neurological signs due to vitamin B$_{12}$ deficiency. The alternative diagnoses include hypothyroidism or folate deficiency. There is a family history of thyroid disease; however, the anaemia is too severe for hypothyroidism. Hypothyroidism or folate deficiency would not explain the neurological signs.

Differential diagnoses of macrocytic anaemia

- Folate deficiency
- Excessive alcohol consumption
- Hypothyroidism
- Certain drugs, e.g. azathioprine, methotrexate
- Primary acquired sideroblastic anaemia and myelodysplastic syndromes

Anaemia results in reduced tissue oxygenation. Symptoms include headache, fatigue, breathlessness and dizziness. There is often pallor of the mucous membranes. Profound vitamin B$_{12}$ deficiency causes a peripheral neuropathy and subacute degeneration of the posterior columns and pyramidal tracts in the spinal cord, causing a sensory loss and increased difficulty walking. The peripheral neuropathy and pyramidal tract involvement produce the combination of absent ankle jerks and upgoing plantars. In its most extreme form it can lead to paraplegia, optic atrophy and dementia.

Vitamin B$_{12}$ is synthesized by micro-organisms and is obtained by ingesting animal or vegetable products contaminated by bacteria. After ingestion, it is bound by intrinsic factor, synthesized by gastric parietal cells, and this complex is then absorbed in the terminal ileum. Vitamin B$_{12}$ deficiency is most commonly of a gastric cause (pernicious anaemia due to an autoimmune atrophic gastritis; total gastrectomy), bacterial overgrowth in the small intestine destroying intrinsic factor, or a malabsorption from the terminal ileum (surgical resection; Crohn's disease).

Pernicious anaemia is the most likely cause of this patient's vitamin B$_{12}$ deficiency. Pernicious anaemia is an autoimmune disease with the production of antibodies that inhibit intrinsic factor binding to vitamin B$_{12}$ in the stomach. Vitamin B$_{12}$ cannot be absorbed in the terminal ileum unless it is bound to the intrinsic factor. In pernicious anaemia, the MCV can rise to 100–140 fL, and oval macrocytes are seen on the blood film. The reticulocyte count is inappropriately low for the degree of anaemia. The white cell count is usually moderately reduced. There is often a mild rise in serum bilirubin giving the patient a 'lemon-yellow' complexion.

A full dietary history should be taken. Vegans who omit all animal products from their diet often have subclinical vitamin B$_{12}$ deficiency. Serum vitamin B$_{12}$ and folate levels should be measured and antibodies to intrinsic factor and parietal cells should be assayed. Intrinsic factor antibodies are virtually specific for pernicious anaemia but are only present in about 50 per cent of cases. Parietal cell antibody is present in 85–90 per cent of patients with pernicious anaemia but can also occur in patients with other causes of atrophic gastritis. A radioactive B$_{12}$ absorption test (Schilling test) distinguishes gastric from intestinal causes of deficiency. Rapid correction of vitamin B$_{12}$ is essential using intramuscular hydroxycobalamin to prevent cardiac failure and further neurological damage.

Differential diagnoses of macrocytic anaemia

- Folate deficiency
- Excessive alcohol consumption
- Hypothyroidism
- Certain drugs (e.g. azathioprine, methotrexate)
- Primary acquired sideroblastic anaemia and myelodysplastic syndromes

KEY POINTS

- Vitamin B_{12} deficiency may occur in strict vegetarians who eat no dairy products.
- Typical neurological signs are position and vibration sense impairment in the legs, absent reflexes and extensor plantars.
- Overenthusiastic blood transfusion should be avoided since it can provoke cardiac failure in vitamin B_{12} deficiency.

INFECTION

History

A 24-year-old man presents to his general practitioner (GP) with a fever. This has been present on and off for 3 days. On the first day he felt a little shaky, but by the third day he felt very unwell with the fever and had a feeling of intense cold with generalized shaking at the same time. He felt very sweaty. The whole episode lasted for 2.5 h, and he felt drained and unwell afterwards. He had lost his appetite.

There is a previous history of hepatitis 4 years earlier, and he had glandular fever at the age of 18 years. He smokes 15–20 cigarettes each day and occasionally smokes marijuana. He denies any intravenous drug abuse. He drinks around 14 units of alcohol each week. He has taken no other medication except for malaria prophylaxis. He denies any homosexual contacts. He has had a number of heterosexual contacts each year but says that all had been with protected intercourse. He had returned from Nigeria 3 weeks earlier and was finishing off his prophylactic malaria regime. He had been in Nigeria for 6 weeks as part of his job working for an oil company and had no illnesses while he was there.

Examination

He looks unwell. His pulse is 94/min; blood pressure is 118/72 mmHg. There are no heart murmurs. There are no abnormalities to find in the respiratory system. In the abdomen there is some tenderness in the left upper quadrant. There are no enlarged lymph nodes.

INVESTIGATIONS

		Normal
Haemoglobin	11.1 g/dL	13.7–17.7 g/dL
Mean corpuscular volume (MCV)	97 fL	80–99 fL
White cell count	9.4×10^9/L	$3.9–10.6 \times 10^9$/L
Neutrophils	6.3×10^9/L	$1.8–7.7 \times 10^9$/L
Lymphocytes	2.9×10^9/L	$1.0–4.8 \times 10^9$/L
Platelets	112×10^9/L	$150–440 \times 10^9$/L
Sodium	134 mmol/L	135–145 mmol/L
Potassium	4.8 mmol/L	3.5–5.0 mmol/L
Urea	4.2 mmol/L	2.5–6.7 mmol/L
Creatinine	74 µmol/L	70–120 µmol/L
Alkaline phosphatase	76 IU/L	30–300 IU/L
Alanine aminotransferase	33 IU/L	5–35 IU/L
Gamma-glutamyl transpeptidase	42 IU/L	11–51 IU/L
Bilirubin	28 mmol/L	3–17 mmol/L
Glucose	4.5 mmol/L	4.0–6.0 mmol/L

Urine: no protein; no blood; no sugar

Questions
- What abnormalities are likely to be present in the blood film?
- What is the most likely diagnosis?
- What would be the appropriate management?

ANSWER 19

There is a raised bilirubin with normal liver enzymes, a mild anaemia with a high normal mean corpuscular volume and a low platelet count. This makes haemolytic anaemia likely. The recent travel to Nigeria raises the possibility of an illness acquired there. The commonest such illness causing a fever in the weeks after return is malaria. The incubation period is usually 12–14 days. Longer incubation periods occur in semi-immune individuals and persons taking inadequate malaria prophylaxis.The mild haemolytic anaemia with a low platelet count would be typical findings. Slight enlargement of liver and spleen may occur after a few days in nonimmune patients with malaria.

The diagnosis should be confirmed by appropriate expert examination of a blood film.

The most important feature in this 24-year-old man is the fever with what sound like rigors. He has no other specific symptoms. He looks unwell, with tachycardia and some tenderness in the left upper quadrant that could be related to splenic enlargement. Malaria prophylaxis is often not taken regularly. Even when it is, it does not provide complete protection against malaria, which should always be suspected in circumstances such as those described here. The risk might be assessed further by finding which parts of Nigeria he spent his time in and whether he remembered mosquito bites. Measures to avoid mosquito bites such as nets, insect repellants and suitable clothing are an important part of prevention.

He has no history of intravenous drug abuse or recent risky sexual contact to suggest HIV infection, although this could not be ruled out. HIV seroconversion can produce a feverish illness but not usually as severe as this. Later in HIV infection an AIDS-related illness would often be associated with a low total lymphocyte count, but this is normal in his case. Other acute viral or bacterial infections are possible but are less likely to explain the abnormal results of some investigations.

The diagnostic test for malaria is staining of a peripheral blood film with a Wright or Giemsa stain. In this case it showed that around 1 per cent of red cells contained parasites. Treatment depends on the likely resistance pattern in the area visited, and up-to-date advice can be obtained by telephone from microbiology departments or tropical disease hospitals. Falciparum malaria is usually treated with quinine sulphate because of widespread resistance to chloroquine. A single dose of Fansidar (pyrimethamine and sulfadoxine) is given at the end of the quinine course for final eradication of parasites. However, there is increasing resistance to quinine, and artemesinin derivatives are increasingly becoming the first-line treatment for falciparum malaria. In severe cases hyponatraemia and hypoglycaemia may occur, and the sodium here is marginally low. Most of the severe complications are associated with *Plasmodium falciparum* malaria. They include cerebral malaria, lung involvement, severe haemolysis and acute renal failure.

 KEY POINTS

- No prophylactic regime is certain to prevent malaria.
- A traveller returning from a malaria endemic region who develops a fever has malaria until proven otherwise.
- Treatment should be guided by advice from tropical disease centres.
- If the malaria species is unknown or the infection mixed, treat as falciparum malaria.

CASE 20: FEVERS AND MALAISE

History

A 54-year-old woman has had diabetes for 40 years controlled on insulin. She also had hypertension treated with amlodipine. Her renal function gradually deteriorated and 18 months earlier she had a deceased donor renal transplant. She had three episodes of rejection treated with increases in her immunosuppression. She had been taking co-trimoxazole but this was discontinued at 12 months post transplant.

She arrived with a fever and malaise which had been present for 5–6 days. She also complained of a non-productive cough for the same period.

Examination

On examination her temperature was 38°C, blood pressure was 132/82, pulse 86/min, respiratory rate was 20/min, saturation 96%. No abnormalities were found in the cardiovascular or respiratory system. There was no tenderness over the transplanted kidney and no lymphadenopathy.

INVESTIGATIONS		
		Normal
Haemoglobin	12.8 g/dL	13.3–17.7 g/dL
Mean corpuscular volume (MCV)	89 fL	80–99 fL
White cell count	8.2 × 10⁹/L	3.9–10.6 × 10⁹/L
Neutrophils	7.6 × 10⁹/L	1.8–7.7 × 10⁹/L
Lymphocytes	0.2 × 10⁹/L	0.6–4.8 × 10⁹/L
Monocytes	0.2 × 10⁹/L	0.6–1.0 × 10⁹/L
Platelets	221 × 10⁹/L	150–440 × 10⁹/L
Sodium	134 mmol/L	135–145 mmol/L
Potassium	4.3 mmol/L	3.5–5.0 mmol/L
Urea	7.2 mmol/L	2.5–6.7 mmol/L
Creatinine	141 µmol/L	70–120 µmol/L
Bilirubin	16 mmol/L	3–17 mmol/L
Alanine transaminase	29 IU/L	5–35 IU/L
Gamma-glutamyl transaminase	53 IU/L	11–51 IU/L
Alkaline phosphatase	251 IU/L	30–300 IU/L

Urinalysis: no protein; no blood
Chest X-ray normal

She was treated with paracetamol and asked to return if there was any deterioration. Three days later she returned with an increase in her fever and cough and a new problem of shortness of breath. On examination her temperature was 38.8°C, blood pressure was 122/78, pulse 90/min, respiratory rate was 26/min, saturation 92%.

Questions
- What is the most likely diagnosis?
- How would you investigate and manage this patient?

ANSWER 20

Fever in a patient who has had a transplant is most often related to a common pathogen, but the presence of immunosuppression raises the possibility of an opportunistic infection. The possibility is higher here because of the increased immunosuppression related to the episodes of rejection.

The symptoms of dry cough and shortness of breath point to a respiratory focus of the infection. Although there was nothing to find on examination of the respiratory system other than the increased respiratory rate and the original chest X-ray was normal, the decrease in oxygen saturation confirms a significant problem with gas exchange in the lung.

The combination of a fever and dry cough with no respiratory signs and increasing hypoxia suggests a diagnosis of *Pneumocystis jiroveci* pneumonia. The chest X-ray may appear normal in the early stages before an increase in diffuse shadowing, with an alveolar filling pattern most marked in the mid and lower zones, often sparing the costophrenic angles (Figure 20.1). This patient was taking co-trimoxazole as prophylaxis against pneumocystis but this was stopped because of a rash increasing the risk of infection.

The first investigation here should be a chest X-ray. Even if sputum is being produced, *Pneumocystis jiroveci* cannot usually be found in the sputum and needs a technique such as sputum induction with hypertonic saline or bronchoscopy with alveolar lavage to sample alveolar contents.

Pneumocystis jiroveci is a fungus previously called *Pneumocystis carinii*. It occurs commonly in the environment but does not cause infection in the absence of immunosuppression. Samples from induced sputum or alveolar lavage are stained with a silver stain, periodic acid Schiff or by immunofluorescence.

Treatment is usually with high dose co-trimoxazole but the previous rash in this patient means that alternative treatments such as dapsone and trimethoprim or clindamycin and primaquine rather than the more toxic alternative of intravenous pentamidine are required. Prednisolone is often used initially in treatment in cases with significant hypoxia.

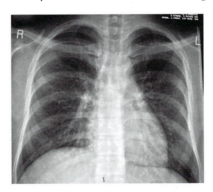

Figure 20.1 Chest X-ray.

 KEY POINTS

- *Pneumocystis jiroveci* is a widespread organism but only causes disease in immuno-suppressed patients.
- Dry cough, fever and breathlessness are common symptoms with tachypnoea and significant hypoxia.
- Diagnosis usually requires sampling of alveolar contents by lavage or sputum induction.

Section 2

GENERAL
SELF-ASSESSMENT CASES

CASE 21: TIREDNESS

History
A 55-year-old man presents to his general practitioner (GP), complaining of lack of energy. He has become increasingly tired over the past 18 months. He works as a solicitor and describes episodes when he has fallen asleep in his office. He is unable to stay awake after 9:30 pm and sleeps through until 7:30 am. He finds it difficult to concentrate at work and has stopped playing his weekly game of tennis. He had an episode of depression 10 years ago related to the break-up of his first marriage. He has no current personal problems. He has had no other major illnesses. His brother developed type 1 diabetes mellitus at the age of 13. On direct questioning, he has noticed that he has become more constipated but denies any abdominal pain or rectal bleeding. He has put on 8 kg in weight over the past year.

Examination
On examination he is overweight. His facial skin is dry and scaly. His pulse is 56/min, regular, and blood pressure is 146/88 mmHg. Examination of his cardiovascular, respiratory and abdominal systems is unremarkable. Neurological examination showed a little proximal weakness.

INVESTIGATIONS

		Normal
Haemoglobin	11.8 g/dL	13.3–17.7 g/dL
Mean corpuscular volume (MCV)	96 fL	80–99 fL
White cell count	4.3 × 10⁹/L	3.9–10.6 × 10⁹/L
Platelets	154 × 10⁹/L	150–440 × 10⁹/L
Sodium	140 mmol/L	135–145 mmol/L
Potassium	4.4 mmol/L	3.5–5.0 mmol/L
Urea	6.4 mmol/L	2.5–6.7 mmol
Creatinine	125 µmol/L	70–120 µmol/L
Glucose	4.7 mmol/L	4.0–6.0 mmol/L
Calcium	2.48 mmol/L	2.12–2.65 mmol/L
Phosphate	1.20 mmol/L	0.8–1.45 mmol/L
Cholesterol	6.4 mmol/L	3.9–6.0 mmol/L
Triglycerides	1.4 mmol/L	0.55–1.90 mmol/L

Urinalysis: nothing abnormal detected (NAD)

Questions
- What is the likely diagnosis?
- How would you further examine, investigate and manage this patient?

ANSWER 21

Fatigue is a very common symptom of both physical and mental illness. The differential diagnosis is extensive and includes cancer, depression, anaemia, renal failure and endocrine diseases. In this case the main differential diagnoses are depression and hypothyroidism. He has a history of depression but currently has no obvious triggers for a further episode of depression. He is not waking early in the morning or having difficulty getting to sleep, which are common biological symptoms of severe depression. There are a number of clues in this case to the diagnosis of hypothyroidism. Insidious onset of fatigue, difficulty concentrating, increased somnolence, constipation and weight gain are features of hypothyroidism. As in this case there may be a family or past medical history of other autoimmune diseases such as type 1 diabetes mellitus, vitiligo or Addison's disease. Hypothyroidism typically presents in the fifth or sixth decade and is about five times more common in women than men. Obstructive sleep apnoea is associated with hypothyroidism and may contribute to daytime sleepiness and fatigue.

On examination the facial appearances and bradycardia are consistent with the diagnosis. Characteristically, patients with overt hypothyroidism have dry, scaly, cold and thickened skin. There may be a malar flush against the background of the pale facial appearance ('strawberries-and-cream appearance'). Scalp hair is usually brittle and sparse, and there may be thinning of the lateral third of the eyebrows. Bradycardia may occur, and the apex beat may be difficult to locate because of the presence of a pericardial effusion. A classic sign of hypothyroidism is the delayed relaxation phase of the ankle jerk. Other neurological syndromes that may occur in association with hypothyroidism include carpal tunnel syndrome, proximal muscle weakness, a cerebellar syndrome or polyneuritis. Patients may present with psychiatric illnesses, including psychoses ('myxoedema madness').

Clues to the diagnosis in the investigations are the mild normochromic, normocytic anaemia, marginally raised creatinine, and hypercholesterolaemia. The anaemia of hypothyroidism is typically normochromic, normocytic or macrocytic; microcytic anaemia may occur if there is menorrhagia. A macrocytic anaemia may represent undiagnosed vitamin B_{12} deficiency. Renal blood flow is reduced in hypothyroidism, and this can cause the creatinine to be slightly above the normal range.

The most severe cases of hypothyroidism present with myxoedema coma, with bradycardia, reduced respiratory rate and severe hypothermia. Typically, shivering is absent.

In this case the thyroid function tests showed thyroid-stimulating hormone (TSH), 73 mU/L (normal range <6 mU/L); free thyroxine (T4), 3 pmol/L (normal range 9–22 pmol/L). The high TSH indicates primary hypothyroidism rather than hypopituitarism. The commonest cause of hypothyroidism is autoimmune thyroiditis, and the patient should have thyroid autoantibodies assayed.

Causes of hypothyroidism

- Panhypopituitarism
- Autoimmune thyroiditis
- Postthyroidectomy
- Postradioiodine treatment for thyrotoxicosis
- Drugs for treatment of hyperthyroidism: carbimazole, propylthiouracil
- Amiodarone, lithium
- Dietary iodine deficiency
- Inherited enzyme defects

Treatment is with T4 at a maintenance dose of 75–200 μg/day. Response is measured clinically and biochemically by the return of TSH to the normal range. Elderly patients or those with coronary heart disease should be started cautiously on T4 because of the risk of precipitating myocardial ischaemia.

KEY POINTS

- Hypothyroidism should be considered in the differential diagnosis of any patient presenting with fatigue.
- A neurological examination should be part of the routine assessment of all such patients.
- Clinical symptoms of hypothyroidism are usually non-specific.
- Hypothyroidism may present in unusual ways, such as psychoses or decreased consciousness level.
- Autoimmune thyroiditis is the commonest cause of hypothyroidism.

History

A 72-year-old man goes to his general practitioner (GP) complaining of painless swelling of both legs, which he first noted approximately 2 months ago. The swelling started at the ankles, but now his legs, thighs and genitals are swollen. His face is puffy in the mornings on getting up. His weight is up by about 10 kg over the previous 3 months. He has noticed that his urine appears to be frothy in the toilet. He has noted gradual increasing shortness of breath but denies any chest pain. He has also developed spontaneous bruising over the past 6 months. He is a retired heavy goods vehicle driver. He had hypertension diagnosed 13 years ago and a myocardial infarction 4 years previously. He lives with his wife and has no children. He continues to smoke 30 cigarettes a day and drinks about 30 units of alcohol a week. His medication consists of atenolol 50 mg once a day.

Examination

On examination there is pitting oedema of the legs, which is present to the level of the sacrum. There is also massive oedema of the penis and scrotum. There is bruising on the forearms and around the eyes. There are no signs of chronic liver disease. His pulse rate is 72/min and regular. Blood pressure is 166/78 mmHg. His jugular venous pressure is raised at 5 cm. His apex beat is not displaced, and auscultation reveals normal heart sounds and no murmurs. There is dullness to percussion and reduced air entry at both lung bases. The liver, spleen and kidneys are not palpable, but ascites is demonstrated by shifting dullness and fluid thrill. Neurological examination is unremarkable.

INVESTIGATIONS

		Normal
Haemoglobin	10.7 g/dL	13.3–17.7 g/dL
Mean corpuscular volume (MCV)	95 fL	80–99 fL
White cell count	4.7 × 10⁹/L	3.9–10.6 × 10⁹/L
Platelets	176 × 10⁹/L	150–440 × 10⁹/L
Sodium	138 mmol/L	135–145 mmol/L
Potassium	4.9 mmol/L	3.5–5.0 mmol/L
Urea	7.4 mmol/L	2.5–6.7 mmol
Creatinine	112 µmol/L	70–120 µmol/L
Glucose	4.7 mmol/L	4.0–6.0 mmol/L
Albumin	16 g/L	35–50 g/L
Cholesterol	15.2 mmol/L	3.9–6.0 mmol/L
Triglycerides	2.7 mmol/L	0.55–1.90 mmol/L

Clotting screen: normal
Urinalysis: +++ protein; no blood

Questions

- What is the cause of this patient's oedema?
- What is the likely underlying diagnosis?
- How would you further examine, investigate and manage this patient?

ANSWER 22

Peripheral oedema may occur due to local obstruction of lymphatic or venous outflow or because of cardiac, renal, pulmonary or liver disease. Unilateral oedema is most likely to be due to a local problem, whereas bilateral leg oedema is usually due to one of the medical conditions listed. Pitting oedema needs to be distinguished from lymphoedema, which is characteristically non-pitting. This is tested by firm pressure with the thumb for approximately 10 s. If the oedema is pitting, an indentation will be present after pressure is removed. This man has a subacute onset of massive pitting oedema. The major differential diagnoses are cardiac failure, renal failure, nephrotic syndrome, right heart failure (cor pulmonale) secondary to chronic obstructive airways disease or decompensated chronic liver disease. The frothy urine is a clue to the diagnosis of nephrotic syndrome and is commonly noted by patients with heavy proteinuria.

On examination there were no clinical signs to suggest chronic liver disease. The jugular venous pressure would be expected to be increased more, and there should have been signs of tricuspid regurgitation (prominent 'v' wave, pansystolic murmur loudest on inspiration) and cardiomegaly if the patient had cor pulmonale or biventricular cardiac failure. The patient has signs of bilateral pleural effusions, which may occur in nephrotic syndrome if there is sufficient fluid retention. The bruising and periorbital purpura are classically seen in patients with nephrotic syndrome secondary to amyloidosis.

The investigations are consistent with the diagnosis of nephrotic syndrome. Nephrotic syndrome is defined by the triad of hypoalbuminaemia (<30 g/L), proteinuria (>3 g/24 h), and hypercholesterolaemia. The normochromic, normocytic anaemia is typical of chronic disease and is a clue to the underlying diagnosis of amyloidosis. Patients with amyloidosis may have raised serum transaminase levels due to liver infiltration by amyloid.

The patient should have a renal biopsy to delineate the cause of the nephrotic syndrome. The principal causes of nephrotic syndrome are listed below. Adults presenting with nephrotic syndrome should have a renal biopsy. The exception is the patient with long-standing diabetes mellitus, with concomitant retinopathy and neuropathy, who almost certainly has diabetic nephropathy.

! Causes of nephrotic syndrome

- Diabetes mellitus
- Minimal change disease
- Focal and segmental glomerulosclerosis
- Membranous nephropathy
- Systemic lupus erythematosus
- HIV infection
- Amyloidosis/myeloma

In this case renal biopsy confirmed the diagnosis of amyloidosis, and staining was positive for lambda light chains. Immunofixation confirmed the presence of a IgG lambda paraprotein in the blood. A bone marrow aspirate showed the presence of an excessive number of plasma cells, consistent with an underlying plasma cell dyscrasia. Patients with amyloidosis should have an echocardiogram to screen for cardiac infiltration, and if the facilities are

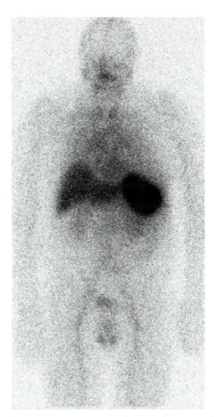

Figure 22.1 Serum amyloid P scan showing uptake predominantly in the spleen.

available, a serum amyloid P scan should be arranged, which assesses the distribution and total body burden of amyloid. An amyloid P scan is shown in Figure 22.1.

The initial treatment of this patient involves fluid and salt restriction and diuretics to reduce the oedema. He should be anticoagulated to reduce the risk of deep vein thrombosis or pulmonary embolus. His hyperlipidaemia should be treated with a statin. Definitive treatment is by chemotherapy supervised by the haematologists to suppress the amyloidogenic plasma cell clone. In younger patients, bone marrow transplantation may be considered. Patients with nephrotic syndrome secondary to amyloidosis usually progress to end-stage renal failure relatively quickly. Death is most commonly due to cardiac involvement.

 KEY POINTS

- Bilateral oedema may be due to cardiac, liver or renal disease.
- All patients presenting with new-onset oedema should have a urinalysis.
- Patients with nephrotic syndrome are at increased risk of pulmonary embolism.

CASE 23: ACUTE DIARRHOEA

History

A 74-year-old woman is admitted from a residential care home with pain in the left iliac fossa. There is no bowel disturbance. She has a history of gastro-oesophageal reflux and is taking lansoprazole daily. She has mild dementia and has lived in the residential home for the last two years. On examination she is tender in the left iliac fossa. A diagnosis of diverticulitis is made and she is treated with cefuroxime intravenously.

She makes a good recovery but on the fifth day of her admission, when she is nearly ready to return to her care home, she has an episode of diarrhoea. The next day she has 4 episodes of watery diarrhoea and complains of crampy abdominal pain.

Examination

On examination her mucous membranes are dry and she has a fever of 38.5°C. She has mild diffuse abdominal tenderness. There is no guarding or rebound tenderness. She has prominent bowel sounds.

INVESTIGATIONS		
		Normal
Haemoglobin	14.2 g/dL	11.7–15.7 g/dL
Mean corpuscular volume (MCV)	87 fL	80–99 fL
White cell count	16.3 × 10⁹/L	3.5–11.0 × 10⁹/L
Platelets	324 × 10⁹/L	150–440 × 10⁹/L
Sodium	134 mmol/L	135–145 mmol/L
Potassium	3.8 mmol/L	3.5–5.0 mmol/L
Urea	9.2 mmol/L	2.5–6.7 mmol/L
Creatinine	189 mmol/L	70–120 µmol/L

Questions

- What is the likely diagnosis?
- How would you further examine, investigate and manage this patient?

ANSWER 23

This patient has developed diarrhoea and abdominal discomfort while in hospital on a course of intravenous broad spectrum antibiotics. This raises the likelihood of infection with *Clostridium difficile*. She has a number of risk factors that make this more likely. She is over 65 years of age, and she lives in a residential care home; 80% of *C. difficile* infections occur in people aged over 65 years since a lower density and fewer species of gut bacteria make them more susceptible to colonisation by *C. difficile*. The use of proton pump inhibitors also increases the risk of colonisation. *C. difficile* spreads by faecal–oral routes and 20% of hospital patients and those in long-term care facilities are colonised with *C. difficile*.

C. difficile is an anaerobic spore forming bacillus, and spores can persist in the environment for some time. Most hospital patients who develop a *C. difficile* infection are being treated with antibiotics and clear guidelines around antibiotic prescribing are integral to limiting *C. difficile* infection.

Stool samples should be obtained and sent for testing from any hospital patient who has unexplained diarrhoea. The initial test generally looks for *C. difficile* toxin and positive tests are confirmed by supplementary tests. Diagnosis depends on the combination of diarrhoea and identification of the toxin or organism, or finding pseudomembranous colitis at colonoscopy.

If *C. difficile* infection is suspected the patient should be isolated, suitable infection control policies should be in place (gloves and apron for contact, hand washing with soap and water). Cases are defined and managed according to severity:

- Mild: mild diarrhoea, normal white cell count, no systemic symptoms
- Moderate: moderate diarrhoea, raised white count $<15 \times 10^9$/L, some systemic symptoms
- Severe: two or more severity measures (temp >38.5C°, in ICU or immunosuppressed, pseudomembranous colitis, toxic megacolon or ileus, colonic dilatation >6 cm on imaging, white count $>15 \times 10^9$/L, creatinine $1.5 \times$ baseline)
- Life threatening: hypotension, ileus or toxic megacolon or CT evidence of severe disease.

Mild or moderate cases are treated with oral metronidazole and moderate to severe cases with oral or parenteral vancomycin.

This woman has evidence of at least severe disease and needs imaging of the bowel with plain abdominal film or CT scan. She should be isolated while results are awaited and treated with fluids and with oral vancomycin.

 KEY POINTS

- *C. difficile* infection should be suspected in any hospital patient who develops diarrhoea.
- A strict antibiotic policy, a high degree of suspicion and good infection control measures all help to reduce problems with *C. difficile* infection.

CASE 24: SHORTNESS OF BREATH ON EXERTION

History

A 23-year-old student presents to her general practitioner (GP) complaining of shortness of breath on exertion. This has developed over the past 10 days, and she is now breathless after walking 50 yards. About 2 weeks ago she had a flu-like illness with generalized muscle aches and fever. She feels extremely tired and has noticed palpitations in association with her breathlessness. In addition she has some discomfort in her anterior chest that is worse on inspiration. Previously she has been extremely fit with no significant past medical history. There is no recent history of foreign travel. She denies substance abuse.

Examination

On examination, her temperature is 37.5°C. Her pulse rate is 120/min and regular. Blood pressure is 90/70 mmHg. Jugular venous pressure is raised at 8 cm. On auscultation there is a gallop rhythm, with a third heart sound. Examination of her chest is unremarkable. Pressure over the sternum causes discomfort. Abdominal and neurological examinations are normal.

> **INVESTIGATIONS**
>
> The GP sends the student to the emergency department, where an electrocardiogram (ECG) and chest X-ray are performed. The ECG shows T-wave flattening globally. The chest X-ray is shown in Figure 24.1.

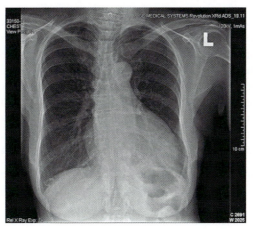

Figure 24.1 Chest X-ray.

Questions

- What is the likely diagnosis?
- How would you further investigate and manage this patient?

ANSWER 24

This patient has viral myocarditis due to Coxsackie B virus. Viruses that can cause myocarditis include Coxsackie B and A, echovirus, adenovirus, influenza, varicella, polio, mumps, rabies, viral hepatitis, rubella, parvovirus B19, Epstein–Barr virus (EBV), cytomegalovirus (CMV), and herpes simplex virus. Myocarditis also may occur during bacteraemia or fungaemia. Rickettsia and diptheria can cause myocarditis. In rural South America acute infection with the protozoan *Trypanosoma cruzi* causes fever, myocarditis and hepatosplenomegaly, and 10–30 years later this can lead to cardiac failure and conduction system defects (Chagas' disease). Cocaine abuse can cause myocarditis and sudden death. Profound hypocalcaemia, hypophosphataemia, and hypomagnaesaemia can all cause myocardial depression.

The clinical picture of myocarditis is non-specific, but common symptoms include myalgia, fatigue, shortness of breath, pericardial pain and palpitations. Myocarditis should be suspected in a young person presenting with new onset cardiac symptoms. There is often a prodromal viral illness affecting the upper respiratory tract or gastrointestinal system. Autoimmune disease such as lupus should be excluded and a careful social history should be taken to exclude alcohol or cocaine abuse. The main clinical signs are those of cardiac failure. A pericardial friction rub may be heard in some patients with myopericarditis. Patients usually have a marked sinus tachycardia disproportionate to the slight fever. ECG usually shows ST segment and T-wave abnormalities. There may be atrial or, more commonly, ventricular arrhythmias or signs of conducting system defects. The chest x-ray may be normal if the myocarditis is mild, but if there is cardiac failure there will be cardiomegaly and pulmonary congestion. The differential diagnoses in this case include hypertrophic cardiomyopathy, pericarditis and myocardial ischaemia.

Cardiac enzymes such as troponin I or T and creatine kinase are raised. Echocardiography should be performed to confirm the diagnosis. Echocardiographic changes may be focal affecting only the right or left ventricle, or global. There is poor contractility of the myocardium. Cardiac enzymes such as troponin I or T and creatine kinase are raised. Cardiac magnetic resonance imaging can detect myocardial oedema and myocyte injury in myocarditis. Coronary angiography may be performed to exclude severe coronary artery disease. Endomyocardial biopsy is considered depending on the course and severity of the condition. Paired serum samples should be taken for antibody titres to Coxsackie B and mumps. Coxsackie virus can be cultured from the throat, stool, blood, myocardium or pericardial fluid.

Bed rest is the treatment for the period of acute viral myocarditis. Diuretics and angiotensin-converting enzyme (ACE) inhibitors are used to treat cardiac failure. Anticoagulation may be required for patients with intracardiac thrombi. There is controversy over treatment with corticosteroids. Corticosteroids tend to be used in patients with a short history, a positive endomyocardial biopsy, and the most severe disease. Most cases are benign and self-limiting, and cardiac function will return to normal. However a minority will develop permanent cardiac damage, leading to dilated cardiomyopathy. Definitive treatment may then involve cardiac transplantation.

KEY POINTS

- The features in favour of the diagnosis of viral myocarditis include the young age of the patient, the preceding acute febrile illness and subsequently the raised serum antibody titres to Coxsackie B.
- It is important to take a history of foreign travel, alcohol intake and substance abuse.
- Outcome in adults is generally good, but a proportion of patients will develop dilated cardiomyopathy.

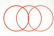

CASE 25: FEVER AND SHORTNESS OF BREATH

History

A 62-year-old man presents to the emergency department complaining of shortness of breath. Four days prior to presentation he felt unwell and complained of muscle aches and headache. The next day he started having rigors, and his wife measured his temperature as 39°C. They thought that he had influenza and he took paracetamol and rested in bed. However his symptoms worsened, and two days later he was complaining of a dry cough and marked shortness of breath. He had also become confused and started having diarrhoea. There is no significant past medical history. He is a non-smoker and drinks 20 units of alcohol a week. Ten days prior to admission he had returned from a coach tour of Spain and Portugal.

Examination

On examination he looks unwell, dehydrated and flushed. His temperature is 39.5°C. He has central cyanosis. His pulse rate is 120/min, and blood pressure is 146/72 mmHg. His respiratory rate is 32/min and oxygen saturation is 86% breathing room air. His trachea is central, and chest expansion is symmetrical. Percussion is reduced at the bases posteriorly, and auscultation reveals bilateral crackles and bronchial breathing in both lower zones posteriorly. His abdomen is diffusely tender, but there is no rigidity or guarding. He is disorientated in time, place and person.

Blood tests, arterial blood gases on air, urinalysis and chest X-ray (Figure 25.1) are shown in the table.

🔍 INVESTIGATIONS		
		Normal
Haemoglobin	15.3 g/dL	13.3–17.7 g/dL
White cell count	10.3×10^9/L	3.9–10.6×10^9/L
Neutrophils	8.9×10^9/L	1.8–7.7×10^9/L
Lymphocytes	0.4×10^9/L	0.6–4.8×10^9/L
Platelets	143×10^9/L	150–440×10^9/L
Sodium	124 mmol/L	135–145 mmol/L
Potassium	4.4 mmol/L	3.5–5.0 mmol/L
Urea	14.4 mmol/L	2.5–6.7 mmol
Creatinine	178 µmol/L	70–120 µmol/L
Glucose	7.7 mmol/L	4.0–6.0 mmol/L
Calcium	1.88 mmol/L	2.12–2.65 mmol/L
Phosphate	1.2 mmol/L	0.8–1.45 mmol/L
C-reactive protein (CRP)	256 mg/L	<5 mg/L
Arterial blood gases on air		
pH	7.38	7.38–7.44
pCO_2	2.7 kPa	4.7–6.0 kPa
pO_2	6.3 kPa	12.0–14.5 kPa

Urinalysis: ++ blood; ++ protein

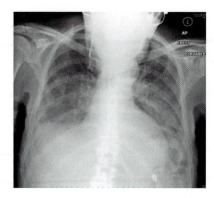

Figure 25.1 Chest X-ray.

Questions

- What is the likely diagnosis?
- How would you further investigate and manage this patient?

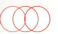

ANSWER 25

This man has signs of pneumonia on clinical examination; this is community acquired pneumonia and the most likely organism given this combination of symptoms and investigations is *Legionella pneumophila* pneumonia. Community-acquired pneumonia is most commonly caused by *Streptococcus pneumoniae* or *Haemophilus influenzae*, but atypical pneumonias (pneumonias caused by 'atypical' organisms such as mycoplasma, legionella and chlamydia without a normal bacterial cell wall) account for about 5–15 per cent of cases. The 4-day prodromal illness is typical of *Legionella* pneumonia (2–10 days) compared to pneumococcal pneumonia, which tends to present abruptly with fever and shortness of breath. *Legionella* infection presents with malaise, myalgia, headache and fever. Patients may develop diarrhoea and abdominal pain. As the illness progresses the patient develops a dry cough, chest pain, shortness of breath and acute confusion. Other potential complications include nephritis, endocarditis and myocarditis. On examination, the patient is usually dehydrated, tachycardic and tachypnoeic, with widespread rhonchi and crackles. The diffuse infiltrates on chest X-ray suggest atypical pneumonia, whereas a lobar pattern tends to occur with streptococcal pneumonia. Hyponatraemia occurs in cases of severe pneumonia and is a poor prognostic factor. Hypocalcaemia is another distinctive biochemical abnormality in this condition. Confusion and raised urea are markers of severity (used in the CURB65 criteria of severity). The high CRP is consistent with a severe infection, and the lymphopenia is a clue to the fact that this patient has an atypical pneumonia. The patient's arterial blood gases showed marked hypoxia with compensatory increased ventilation producing the low $PaCO_2$. This patient presumably acquired his infection while on holiday in Spain or Portugal. *Legionella* outbreaks have often been due to infected water tanks in warm climates in institutions such as hotels and hospitals.

This man is acutely unwell and needs to be admitted to a high-dependency unit. He needs to receive a high concentration of inspired oxygen and intravenous fluids to correct his dehydration. He may require ventilatory support. He should be started on intravenous antibiotics immediately. These should cover the common community-acquired pneumonias until the precise microbiological diagnosis is obtained and the antibiotics can then be rationalized. A standard combination is cefuroxime and clarithromycin. Blood cultures should be sent and blood sent to screen for antibodies to atypical organisms and influenza. Ten to fourteen days later a further blood sample should be sent, and a fourfold rise in antibody titre is evidence of current infection. A faster diagnosis is made by testing broncheoalveolar lavage fluid, blood and urine for the presence of *Legionella* antigen.

 KEY POINTS

- *Legionella* is one of the atypical causes of pneumonia.
- It should be suspected if there is an outbreak in an institution or if a case of pneumonia fails to respond to antibiotics.
- *Legionella* pneumonia has a 2- to 10-day prodromal period.
- Lymphopenia, evidence of nephritis, and a diffuse pattern of infiltrates on chest X-ray are other clues to the diagnosis.

CASE 26: LOIN PAIN AND HAEMATURIA

History

A 46-year-old woman presents to the emergency department with a 2-day history of right-sided loin pain and macroscopic haematuria. The pain is continuous and dull in character. Over the past 10 years she has had previous episodes of loin pain that have occurred on both sides and resolved spontaneously over a few days. She has never passed any stones. She was noted to be mildly hypertensive during her three pregnancies. She has no other significant medical history. Her father died of a subarachnoid haemorrhage, aged 48 years. Her father's brother has had a kidney transplant. She has no siblings. Her three children, aged 17, 14 and 10 years, are well. She works as a teacher and neither smokes nor drinks alcohol.

Examination

On examination she is afebrile. Her pulse is regular at 76/min, and her blood pressure is 135/105 mmHg. Examination of the cardiovascular and respiratory systems is otherwise unremarkable. On palpation of her abdomen, ballottable masses are palpable in each flank. The right-sided mass is tender to palpation. Percussion note is resonant over the masses. Neurological examination is normal. Funduscopy shows arteriovenous nipping and silver-wiring of the retinal vessels.

🔍 INVESTIGATIONS

		Normal
Haemoglobin	14.3 g/dL	11.7–15.7 g/dL
White cell count	5.2×10^9/L	3.5–11.0×10^9/L
Platelets	206×10^9/L	150–440×10^9/L
Sodium	138 mmol/L	135–145 mmol/L
Potassium	4.3 mmol/L	3.5–5.0 mmol/L
Urea	10.2 mmol/L	2.5–6.7 mmol/L
Creatinine	146 µmol/L	70–120 µmol/L
Albumin	42 g/L	35–50 g/L

Urinalysis: + protein; +++ blood
Urine microscopy: >200 red cells; 10 white cells; no organisms
Abdominal X-ray: no intra-abdominal calcification seen

Questions

- What is the diagnosis?
- How would you proceed to manage and investigate this patient?

ANSWER 26

This patient has autosomal dominant polycystic kidney disease (ADPKD). She has macroscopic haematuria, hypertension and impaired renal function. The palpable abdominal masses in both flanks have the characteristic features of enlarged kidneys. They are ballottable and resonant to percussion because of overlying bowel. The other principal causes for palpable kidneys are renal cell carcinoma and massive hydronephrosis. Rest is the best management for cyst bleeding. Gross haematuria rarely lasts for more than a week.

ADPKD is the most common inherited renal disease, occurring in approximately 1:600 to 1:1000 individuals. Although the name 'ADPKD' is derived from renal manifestations of cyst growth leading to enlarged kidneys and renal failure, this is a systemic disorder manifested by the presence of hepatic cysts, diverticular disease, inguinal hernias, mitral valve prolapse, intracranial aneurysms and hypertension. Flank pain is the most common symptom and may be caused by cyst rupture, cyst infection or renal calculi. Macroscopic haematuria due to cyst haemorrhage occurs commonly and usually resolves spontaneously. Renal calculi occur in approximately 20 per cent of ADPKD patients (most commonly uric acid stones). Hypertension occurs early in the course of this disease, affecting 60% of patients with normal renal function. Approximately 50% of ADPKD patients will develop end-stage renal failure.

Although it is not known if this patient's father had renal disease, it is highly likely that he had ADPKD and an associated ruptured berry aneurysm as the cause for his subarachnoid haemorrhage. The patient's uncle required a renal transplant. The pattern of inheritance in this family is consistent with an autosomal dominant trait.

Ultrasound is the preferred initial screening technique as it is cheap, non-invasive and rapid. It detects cysts as small as 0.5 cm. For a certain diagnosis, there should be at least three renal cysts with at least one cyst in each kidney. Computed tomography (CT) and magnetic resonance imaging (MRI) are more sensitive techniques for detecting smaller cysts. Ultrasound in this patient shows the typical appearance of multiple cysts (black areas) surrounded by thickened walls (Figure 26.1). She should be referred to a nephrologist for long-term follow-up of her renal failure, and plans should be made for renal replacement therapy. She needs to have effective blood pressure control with diastolic pressure less than 85 mmHg to retard the progression of her renal failure. Clinical trials are starting of vasopressin receptor antagonists, which show promise at inhibiting cyst growth.

She should have MRI angiography to exclude an intracranial aneurysm. This is not advocated for all ADPKD patients but is indicated for those patients with a positive family history of aneurysm rupture. The patient's children should have their blood pressure checked and later be screened by ultrasound. By age 30 years, 90% of ADPKD patients will have cysts detectable by ultrasound.

Ninety per cent of ADPKD patients have mutations in the *ADPKD1* gene. This gene encodes for the protein polycystin, which is a membrane glycoprotein that probably mediates cell–cell or cell–matrix interactions. Most remaining patients have mutations in the *ADPKD2* gene, which codes for polycystin-2, which has structural homology to polycystin and to calcium channels. *ADPKD1* patients generally have an earlier age of onset of hypertension and development of renal failure as compared to *ADPKD2* patients.

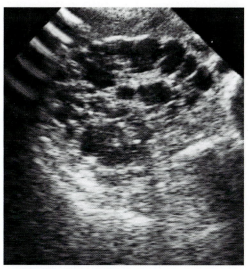

Figure 26.1 Renal ultrasound demonstrating multiple cysts.

 KEY POINTS

- Patients with ADPKD are often asymptomatic.
- ADPKD patients may present with loin pain or haematuria.
- ADPKD is the commonest familial cause of renal failure.
- ADPKD is the most likely cause of bilateral renal masses.
- Family members who may have ADPKD should be advised to have their blood pressure measured and a renal ultrasound.

CASE 27: JOINT PAINS

History

A 38-year-old woman presents to her general practitioner (GP) complaining of pains in her joints. She has noticed these pains worsening over several months. Her joints are most stiff on waking in the mornings. The joints that are most painful are the small joints of the hands and feet. The pain is relieved by diclofenac tablets. She feels tired and has lost 4 kg in weight over 3 months. She has had no previous serious illnesses. She is married with two children and works as a legal secretary. She is a non-smoker and drinks alcohol only occasionally. Her only medication is diclofenac.

Examination

On examination she looks pale and is clinically anaemic. Her proximal interphalangeal joints and metacarpophalangeal joints are swollen and painful, with effusions present. Her metatarsophalangeal joints are also tender. Physical examination is otherwise normal.

INVESTIGATIONS		
		Normal
Haemoglobin	8.9 g/dL	11.7–15.7 g/dL
Mean corpuscular volume (MCV)	87 fL	80–99 fL
White cell count	7.2 × 10⁹/L	3.5–11.0 × 10⁹/L
Platelets	438 × 10⁹/L	150–440 × 10⁹/L
Erythrocyte sedimentation rate (ESR)	78 mm/h	<10 mm/h
Sodium	141 mmol/L	135–145 mmol/L
Potassium	3.9 mmol/L	3.5–5.0 mmol/L
Urea	6.9 mmol/L	2.5–6.7 mmol/L
Creatinine	125 µmol/L	70–120 µmol/L
Glucose	4.6 mmol/L	4.0–6.0 mmol/L
Albumin	33 g/L	35–50 g/L

Urinalysis: no protein; no blood; no glucose

Questions

- What is the diagnosis, and what are the major differential diagnoses?
- How would you investigate and manage this patient?

ANSWER 27

This patient has symptoms and signs typical of early rheumatoid arthritis. Rheumatoid arthritis is a chronic, systemic inflammatory disorder principally affecting joints in a peripheral symmetrical distribution. The peak incidence is between 35 and 55 years in women and 40 and 60 years in men. It is a disease with a long course with exacerbations and remissions. The acute presentation may occur over the course of a day and be associated with fever and malaise. More commonly, as in this case, it presents insidiously, and this group has a worse prognosis. Rheumatoid arthritis characteristically affects proximal interphalangeal, metacarpophalangeal and wrist joints in the hands and metatarsophalangeal joints, ankles, knees and cervical spine.

Early morning stiffness of the joints is typical of rheumatoid arthritis. As the disease progresses, damage to cartilage, bone and tendons leads to the characteristic deformities of this condition. Extra-articular features include rheumatoid nodules, vasculitis causing cutaneous nodules and digital gangrene, scleritis, pleural effusions, diffuse pulmonary fibrosis, pulmonary nodules, obliterative bronchiolitis, pericarditis and splenomegaly (Felty's syndrome). There is usually a normochromic, normocytic anaemia and raised ESR, as seen here. The degree of anaemia and ESR roughly correlates with disease activity. In this case the raised creatinine is probably due to the use of diclofenac. Non-steroidal anti-inflammatory drugs (NSAIDs) reduce glomerular filtration rate in all patients. Rarely they can cause an acute interstitial nephritis. In patients with long-standing rheumatoid arthritis, renal infiltration by amyloid may occur.

> **! Differential diagnosis of an acute symmetrical polyarthritis**
>
> - *Osteoarthritis*: characteristically affects the distal interphalangeal as well as proximal interphalangeal and first metacarpophalangeal joints.
> - *Rheumatoid arthritis*.
> - *Systemic lupus erythematosus*: usually causes a mild, flitting, non-erosive arthritis.
> - *Gout*: usually starts as monoarthritis.
> - *Seronegative arthritides*: ankylosing spondylitis, psoriasis, Reiter's disease. These usually cause asymmetrical arthritis affecting medium and larger joints as well as the sacroiliac and distal interphalangeal joints.
> - *Acute viral arthritis (e.g. rubella)*: resolves completely.

This patient should be referred to a rheumatologist for further investigation and management. The affected joints should be X-rayed. If there has been joint damage, the X-rays will show subluxation, juxta-articular osteoporosis, loss of joint space and bony erosions. A common site for erosions to be found in early rheumatoid arthritis is the fifth metatarsophalangeal joint (arrowed in Figure 27.1). Blood tests should be taken for rheumatoid factor (present in rheumatoid arthritis) and anti-DNA antibodies (present in systemic lupus erythematosus). This patient should be given NSAIDs for analgesia and to reduce joint stiffness to allow her to continue her secretarial work. Disease-modifying drugs such as hydroxychloroquine, sulfasalazine, methotrexate, or leflunomide should be considered unless the patient settles easily on NSAIDs. Addition of an anti-tumour necrosis factor (TNF) antibody is considered where the disease fails to come under control with methotrexate.

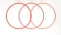

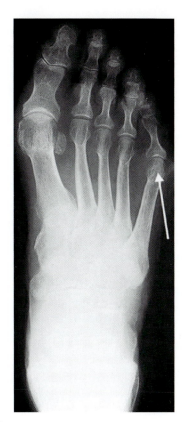

Figure 27.1 X-ray of the foot.

 KEY POINTS

- Rheumatoid arthritis tends to spare the distal interphalangeal joints.
- Systemic symptoms of rheumatoid arthritis may precede the joint symptoms.
- Anaemia and ESR correlate with disease activity.
- NSAIDs may adversely affect renal function.

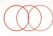

CASE 28: CHRONIC CHEST PAIN

History

A 30-year-old woman is complaining of chest pain. This had been present for 2 years on and off. The pain settled for a period of 6 months, but it has returned over the last 10 months and she is worried that the pain originates in her heart. The pain usually starts on the left side of the chest, radiating to the left axilla. She describes it as a tight or gripping pain that lasts for anything from 5 to 30 min at a time. It can come on at any time and is often related to exercise, but it has occurred at rest, particularly in the evenings. The pain is usually associated with shortness of breath. It makes her stop whatever she is doing, and she often feels faint or dizzy with the pain. Occasionally palpitations come on after the start of the pain. Detailed questioning about the palpitations indicates that they are a sensation of a strong but steady heartbeat.

In her medical history, she had her appendix removed at the age of 15 years. At the age of 24 years she was investigated for an irregular bowel habit and abdominal pain, but no specific diagnosis was reached. These symptoms still trouble her. She has seasonal rhinitis. Two years ago she visited a chemist and had her cholesterol level measured; the result was 4.1 mmol/L. In her family history her grandfather died of a myocardial infarction, a year previously, aged 77 years. Several members of her family have hay fever or asthma. She works as a medical secretary. She is married and has no children.

Examination

On examination, she has a blood pressure of 102/65 mmHg and pulse of 78/min, which is regular. The heart sounds are normal. There is some tenderness on the left side of the chest, to the left of the sternum and in the left submammary area. The respiratory rate is 22/min. No abnormalities were found on examination of the lungs. She is tender in the left iliac fossa.

 INVESTIGATIONS

- Her electrocardiogram (ECG) is shown in Figure 28.1.
- She asked to be referred for a coronary arteriogram to rule out significant coronary artery disease.

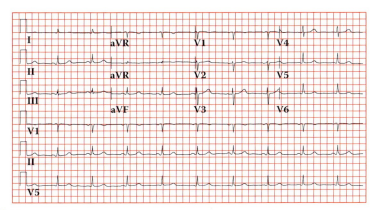

Figure 28.1 Electrocardiogram.

Question

- What should be done?

ANSWER 28

The ECG shown is normal. The pain does not have the characteristics of ischaemic heart disease in that it has a variable relation to exercise, starts on the left side and lasts for up to 30 min. Based on the information given here it would be reasonable to explore her anxieties and to reassure the patient that this is very unlikely to represent coronary artery disease and to subsequently assess the effects of that reassurance. It may well be that she is anxious about the death of her grandfather from ischaemic heart disease. He may have had symptoms before his death that were related to her anxieties. From a risk point of view her grandfather's death at the age of 77 with no other affected relatives is not a relevant risk factor. She has expressed anxiety already by having her cholesterol measured (and found to be normal).

She has a history that is suspicious of irritable bowel syndrome with persistent pain, irregular bowel habit and normal investigations. Ischaemic chest pain is usually central and generally reproducible with the same stimuli. The associated shortness of breath may reflect overventilation coming on with the pain and giving her dizziness and palpitations.

The characteristics of the pain and associated shortness of breath should be explored further. Asthma can sometimes be described as tightness or pain in the chest, and she has seasonal rhinitis and a family history of asthma. Gastrointestinal causes of pain such as reflux oesophagitis are unlikely in view of the site and relationship on occasions to exercise. The length of the history excludes other causes of acute chest pain, such as pericarditis. Chronic hyperventilation or psychogenic dyspnoea may be detected from a low $PaCO_2$ often with compensatory low bicarbonate level and an abnormal breathing pattern, often with sighing breaths. However, it is important to remember that patients with psychogenic dyspnoea may develop other medical problems.

The problem of embarking on tests is that there is no simple screening test that can definitively rule out significant coronary artery disease. Too many investigations may reinforce her belief in her illness, and false-positive findings do occur and may exacerbate her anxieties. However, if the patient could not be simply reassured, it might be appropriate to proceed with an exercise stress test or a thallium scan to look for areas of reversible ischaemia on exercise or other stress. If this is normal she can then be reassured strongly with confidence. A coronary arteriogram would not be appropriate without other information to indicate a higher degree of risk of coronary artery disease.

 KEY POINTS

- Ischaemic heart disease characteristically causes central rather than left-sided chest pain.
- The resting ECG may show signs of ischaemia or previous infarction but is not a very sensitive test for ischaemic heart disease.

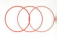

CASE 29: OVERDOSE?

History

A 30-year-old woman is brought to the emergency department at 2 pm by her husband. He is worried that she has taken some tablets in an attempt to harm herself. She has a history suggestive of depression since the birth of her son 3 months earlier. She has been having some counselling since that time but has not been on any medication. The previous evening about 10 pm, she told her husband that she was going to take some pills and locked herself in the bathroom. Two hours later he persuaded her to come out, and she said that she had not taken anything. They went to bed, but he has brought her now because she has complained of a little nausea, and he is worried that she might have taken something when she was in the bathroom. The only tablets in the house were aspirin, paracetamol and temazepam, which he takes occasionally for insomnia.

She complains of a little nausea, although she has not vomited. She has had a little abdominal discomfort. There is no relevant previous medical or family history of note. She worked as a social worker until 30 weeks of the pregnancy.

Examination

On examination she is mentally alert. She says that she feels sad. Her pulse is 76/min, blood pressure is 124/78 mmHg, and respiratory rate is 16/min. There is some mild abdominal tenderness in the upper abdomen, but nothing else abnormal is found.

INVESTIGATIONS		Normal
Haemoglobin	12.7 g/dL	11.7–15.7 g/dL
Mean corpuscular volume (MCV)	87 fL	80–99 fL
White cell count	6.8×10^9/L	$3.5–11.0 \times 10^9$/L
Platelets	230×10^9/L	$150–440 \times 10^9$/L
Prothrombin time	18 s	10–14 s
Sodium	139 mmol/L	135–145 mmol/L
Potassium	3.8 mmol/L	3.5–5.0 mmol/L
Urea	4.6 mmol/L	2.5–6.7 mmol/L
Creatinine	81 µmol/L	70–120 µmol/L
Alkaline phosphatase	88 IU/L	30–300 IU/L
Alanine aminotransferase (AAT)	37 IU/L	5–35 IU/L
Gamma-glutamyl transpeptidase	32 IU/L	11–51 IU/L
Glucose	5.1 mmol/L	4.0–6.0 mmol/L

Question

- What should the management be now?

ANSWER 29

It is not evident from the history that the patient herself has been asked about any tablets or other agents she has taken. This would be an important area to be sure about. Of the three agents mentioned, the only one likely to be relevant is paracetamol. Aspirin and temazepam would be likely to produce more symptoms in less than 14 h if they have been taken in significant quantity. However, the salicylate level should certainly be measured; in this case it was not raised. In the absence of drowsiness at this time, it is not necessary to consider temazepam any further.

Paracetamol overdose causes hepatic and renal damage and can lead to death from acute liver failure. The severity of paracetamol poisoning is dose related, with a dose of 15 g being serious in most patients. Patients with pre-existing liver disease and those with a high alcohol intake may be susceptible to smaller overdoses.

The only significant abnormality on the blood tests is a slightly high prothrombin time and minimally raised AAT. The prothrombin time increase (expressed alternatively as the international normalized ratio or INR) is a signal that a paracetamol overdose is likely. It is often the first test to become abnormal when there is liver damage from paracetamol overdose. If the INR is abnormal at 24 h, then a significant problem is very likely. There are few symptoms in the first 24 h except perhaps nausea, vomiting and abdominal discomfort. This may be associated with tenderness over the liver. The liver function tests usually become abnormal after the first 24 h. Maximum liver damage, as assessed by raised liver enzymes and INR, occurs at days 3–4 after overdose. Acute liver failure may develop between days 3 and 5, and renal failure occurs in about 25% of patients with severe hepatic damage. Rarely, renal failure can occur without serious liver damage.

The paracetamol level should be measured urgently; it was found to be high. The evidence of early liver damage from the INR would in itself suggest that treatment with acetylcysteine would be appropriate. The earlier this is used the better, but it is certainly still worthwhile 16 h after the ingestion. In this case, a level of paracetamol of 64 mg/L confirmed that treatment was appropriate, and that the risk of severe liver damage was high. Further advice can always be obtained by ringing one of the national poison information services. The electrolyte, renal and liver function tests and clotting studies should be monitored carefully over the first few days and referral to a liver unit considered if there is marked liver dysfunction. Patients with fulminant hepatic failure are considered for urgent liver transplantation.

The other areas that need to be addressed in this case are the mental state and the safety and care of her son and any other children. This is a serious drug overdose. She should be seen by a psychiatrist or other appropriately trained health worker. The question of any possible risk to the baby should be evaluated before she returns home.

 KEY POINTS

- Intravenous acetylcysteine and oral methionine are effective treatments for paracetamol overdose if started early enough.
- Paracetamol levels can be used to predict problems and guide treatment if the time since overdose is known.
- Paracetamol overdose should be suspected in any patient admitted with deranged liver function tests and clotting if no obvious alternative cause is apparent.

CASE 30: AMENORRHOEA

History

A 23-year-old actress presents to her general practitioner (GP) complaining that she has not had a menstrual period for 5 months. She started having periods aged 13 years, and previously they had been regular. On direct questioning she states that she has lost 8 kg in weight over the past year, although she says her appetite is good. She has had no serious medical illnesses. Currently she is out of work. She split up from her boyfriend 1 year ago. She drinks 10 units of alcohol per week and is a non-smoker. She is taking no regular medication.

Examination

She has lost muscle mass, especially on her limbs and buttocks. She is 1.7 m (5 ft 9 in.) tall and weighs only 41 kg. She has excessive hair growth over her cheeks, neck and forearms. Her pulse rate is 52/min and regular; blood pressure is 96/60 mmHg. Examination is otherwise normal.

INVESTIGATIONS

		Normal
Haemoglobin	15.2 g/dL	11.7–15.7 g/dL
Mean corpuscular volume (MCV)	84 fL	80–99 fL
White cell count	4.1×10^9/L	$3.5–11.0 \times 10^9$/L
Platelets	365×10^9/L	$150–440 \times 10^9$/L
Sodium	136 mmol/L	135–145 mmol/L
Potassium	2.9 mmol/L	3.5–5.0 mmol/L
Chloride	90 mmol/L	95–105 mmol/L
Bicarbonate	33 mmol/L	24–30 mmol/L
Urea	4.2 mmol/L	2.5–6.7 mmol/L
Creatinine	43 µmol/L	70–120 µmol/L
Glucose	5.6 mmol/L	4.0–6.0 mmol/L
Albumin	41 g/L	35–50 g/L

Questions

- What is the clinical diagnosis?
- How should this patient be investigated and managed?

ANSWER 30

This picture of loss of menstruation (secondary amenorrhoea), weight loss (to a body mass index [BMI] of 14.0) and hypokalaemic, hypochloraemic metabolic alkalosis fits well with a diagnosis of anorexia nervosa. This is a disorder usually of teenagers or young adults characterized by severe weight loss, a disorder of body image (the patients perceiving themselves as fat despite being objectively thin) and amenorrhoea (or, in men, loss of libido or potency). It is commoner in women than men. Often sufferers from this condition work in a profession where personal image is very important (e.g. models, actresses, ballet dancers), and there may be a trigger of an emotional upset such as break-up of a relationship or failure in important examinations. Patients may abuse purgatives or diuretics or cause self-induced vomiting. Some patients exhibit the bulimic behaviour of recurrent bouts of overeating and self-induced vomiting. Patients often deny that they are ill or that they need medical attention. There is marked wasting with obvious bony prominences. The skin is dry with growth of lanugo hair over the neck, cheeks and limbs, as in this woman. There is usually sinus bradycardia and hypotension. There may be calluses on the dorsum of the hand (Russell's sign) due to pressure of teeth on the skin whilst inducing vomiting. There is often parotid gland swelling with discoloured teeth due to the effect of gastric acid causing loss of dental enamel. Severe physical complications include proximal myopathy, cardiomyopathy and peripheral neuropathy.

> **!** **Major causes of secondary amenorrhoea**
>
> - Hypothalmic/pituitary pathology (e.g. hypopituitarism, hyperprolactinaemia)
> - Gonadal failure (e.g. autoimmune ovarian failure, polycystic ovaries)
> - Uterine damage from previous postpartum haemorrhage or instrumentation.
> - Adrenal disease (e.g. Cushing's disease)
> - Thyroid disorders (e.g. both hypothyroidism and hyperthyroidism)
> - Severe chronic illnesses (e.g. cancer, chronic renal failure)

A number of interrelated mechanisms cause the metabolic alkalosis in this patient. The vomiting causes a net loss of hydrogen and chloride ions, causing alkalosis and hypochloraemia. The loss of fluid by vomiting leads to a contracted plasma volume with consequent secondary hyperaldosteronism to conserve sodium and water, but with renal loss of potassium due to its secretion in preference to sodium and the fact that fewer hydrogen ions are available for secretion by the renal tubules. These events combine to give the typical picture of alkalosis with low chloride and raised bicarbonate in the blood; urine containing excess potassium and very little chloride. Measurement of 24 h urinary chloride excretion is helpful. A low urinary chloride excretion (<10 mmol/day) implies vomiting, whereas higher values suggest diuretic abuse.

This patient should be referred to a unit with a special interest in eating disorders. Other serious physical illnesses should be excluded with the appropriate investigations. Plasma levels of luteinizing hormone (LH), follicle-stimulating hormone (FSH) and oestrogens will be low. Often such patients are admitted for several weeks in an attempt to make them gain weight. This involves a high-calorie diet with support from the medical and nursing team. Supportive psychotherapy tackles the patient's disordered perception of personal body image.

> **KEY POINTS**
>
> - Anorexia nervosa is a common cause of amenorrhoea in young women.
> - Hypokalaemic metabolic alkalosis is the characteristic metabolic abnormality.
> - Anorexia nervosa may be associated with abuse of diuretics or purgatives.

CASE 31: PAIN IN THE BACK

History

A 75-year-old woman presents to her general practitioner (GP) complaining of severe back pain. This developed suddenly a week previously after carrying a heavy suitcase at the airport. The pain is persistent and in her lower back. She has had increasing problems with back pain over the past 10 years, and her family has commented on how stooped her posture has become. Her height has decreased by around 10 cm over this period. Her past medical history is notable for severe chronic asthma. She takes courses of oral corticosteroids often for several months three to four times a year, and uses steroid inhalers on a regular basis. She fell 2 years ago and sustained a Colles' fracture to her left wrist. Her menopause occurred at 42 years. She smokes 30 cigarettes a day and drinks four bottles of wine a week.

Examination

She has thoracic kyphosis. She is tender over the L4 vertebra. She has some abdominal striae and a number of bruises on her arms and thighs. She is not anaemic, and examination is otherwise unremarkable.

INVESTIGATIONS		
		Normal
Haemoglobin	11.9 g/dL	11.7–15.7 g/dL
Mean corpuscular volume (MCV)	103 fL	80–99 fL
White cell count	6.2 × 10⁹/L	3.5–11.0 × 10⁹/L
Platelets	358 × 10⁹/L	150–440 × 10⁹/L
Erythrocyte sedimentation rate (ESR)	8 mm/h	<10 mm/h
Sodium	143 mmol/L	135–145 mmol/L
Potassium	4.9 mmol/L	3.5–5.0 mmol/L
Urea	5.9 mmol/L	2.5–6.7 mmol/L
Creatinine	102 µmol/L	70–120 µmol/L
Calcium	2.42 mmol/L	2.12–2.65 mmol/L
Phosphate	1.26 mmol/L	0.8–1.45 mmol/L
Alkaline phosphatase	156 IU/L	30–300 IU/L

X-ray of the lumbar spine is shown in Figure 31.1.

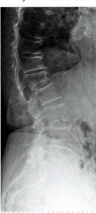

Questions
- What is the likely diagnosis?
- How would you manage this patient?

Figure 31.1 X-ray of the lumbar spine.

ANSWER 31

This woman has a kyphosis, localised back pain and radiological evidence of fracture indicating a likely diagnosis of vertebral collapse secondary to osteoporosis. The loss of height is typical and is usually noted more by others than the patient. The back pain is due to collapse of the vertebrae. This can occur spontaneously or in association with a recognized stress, such as lifting or carrying a heavy load. Examination confirms loss of trunk height, thoracic kyphosis and proximity of the ribs to the iliac crest.

> **! The differential diagnoses of osteoporosis**
>
> - Multiple myeloma
> - Metastatic carcinoma, particularly from the prostate, breast, bronchus, thyroid and kidney
> - Osteomalacia
> - Hyperparathyroidism
> - Steroid therapy or Cushing's syndrome

This patient has several risk factors for osteoporosis. Firstly she is aged 75 years, and ageing is associated with bone loss. Secondly she has been postmenopausal for over 30 years. Premenopausal ovarian production of oestrogens helps to preserve bone mass. Thirdly she has been on oral and inhaled corticosteroids for her asthma for years. Finally, excess alcohol intake may also be a factor. Her red cells are macrocytic, which is consistent with heavy alcohol intake. Alcohol can lead to an increased incidence of falls and fractures. She has no clinical evidence of thyrotoxicosis or hypopituitarism, which can cause osteoporosis.

This woman should have blood tests to exclude myeloma, cancer and metabolic bone disease. Patients with myeloma are anaemic with a raised ESR and a monoclonal paraprotein band on serum protein electrophoresis. In contrast to metabolic bone diseases biochemical measurements (serum calcium, alkaline phosphatase and parathormone [PTH]) in osteoporosis are normal. She should have plain X-rays of her spine. Collapse of the vertebral body will manifest as irregular anterior wedging affecting some vertebrae and not others (L1 and L4). A dual-energy X-ray absorptiometry (DEXA) scan can be performed to assess the severity of the osteoporosis, but treatment is indicated anyway with a fracture at this age.

She should have her dose of corticosteroids reduced to the minimum required to control her asthmatic symptoms, using the inhaled routes as much as possible. Inhaled steroids can cause bruising and systemic effects in prolonged high dose but rarely cause osteoporosis and are considerably safer than oral corticosteroids.She should be started on calcium and vitamin D supplements and a bisphosphonate to try to reduce her bone loss. Oestrogen-based hormone replacement therapy is only used for symptoms associated with menopause because of the increased incidence of thromboembolism and endometrial carcinoma. Other possible treatments for osteoporosis include strontium and parathyroid hormone.

> **🔑 KEY POINTS**
>
> - Osteoporosis is common in the elderly.
> - Bone loss is more rapid in women than men.
> - DEXA scan is the method of choice for screening for osteoporosis.
> - There are increasingly effective treatments available for the treatment of osteoporosis.

CASE 32: ABDOMINAL PAIN

History

A 31-year-old woman has a 6-year history of abdominal pain and bloating. She has had an irregular bowel habit with periods of increased bowel actions up to four times a day and periods of constipation. Opening her bowels tends to relieve the pain, which has been present in both iliac fossae at different times. She had similar problems around the age of 17 years, which led to time off school. She thinks that her pains are made worse after eating citrus fruits and after some vegetables and wheat. She has tried to exclude these from her diet with some temporary relief, but overall there has been no change in the symptoms over the 6 years. One year previously she was seen in a gastroenterology clinic and had a sigmoidoscopy, which was normal. She found the procedure very uncomfortable and developed similar symptoms of abdominal pain during the procedure. She is anxious about the continuing pain but is not keen to have a further endoscopy.

She has a history of occasional episodes of headache, which have been diagnosed as migraine, and has irregular periods with troublesome period pains but no other relevant medical history. She is a non-smoker who does not drink alcohol. Her paternal grandmother died at age 64 years of carcinoma of the colon. Her parents are alive and well. She works as a secretary.

Examination

Examination of the cardiovascular and respiratory systems is normal. She has a palpable, rather tender, colon in the left iliac fossa.

INVESTIGATIONS

		Normal
Haemoglobin	11.9 g/dL	11.7–15.7 g/dL
Mean corpuscular volume (MCV)	84 fL	80–99 fL
White cell count	5.3 × 10⁹/L	3.5–11.0 × 10⁹/L
Platelets	244 × 10⁹/L	150–440 × 10⁹/L
Erythrocyte sedimentation rate (ESR)	8 mm/h	<10 mm/h
Sodium	138 mmol/L	135–145 mmol/L
Potassium	4.4 mmol/L	3.5–5.0 mmol/L
Urea	4.2 mmol/L	2.5–6.7 mmol/L
Creatinine	89 µmol/L	70–120 µmol/L
Glucose	4.6 mmol/L	4.0–6.0 mmol/L

Question

- What is the most likely diagnosis, and what investigations should be performed?

ANSWER 32

The pattern of the pain, the absence of physical signs, normal investigations and reproduction of the pain during sigmoidoscopy all make it likely that this is irritable bowel syndrome (IBS). This is a very common condition accounting for a large number of referrals to gastroenterology clinics. IBS is often episodic, with variable periods of relapse and remission. Periods of frequent defaecation alternate with periods of relative constipation. Relapses are often associated with periods of stress. In IBS it is common to have a history of other conditions, such as migraine and menstrual irregularity. Under the age of 40 years with a history of 6 years of similar problems, it would be reasonable to accept the diagnosis and reassure the patient. However, the family history of carcinoma of the colon raises the possibility of a condition such as familial polyposis coli. The family history, the circumstances of the grandmother's death and the patient's feelings about this should be explored further. Anxiety about the family history might contribute to the patient's own symptoms or her presentation at this time. If there are living family members with polyposis coli, DNA probing may be used to identify family members at high risk. If any doubt remains in this woman it would be sensible to proceed to a barium enema or a colonoscopy to rule out any significant problems.

The diagnosis of IBS relies on the exclusion of other significant conditions, such as inflammatory bowel disease, diverticular disease or large-bowel malignancy. In patients under the age of 40 years it is usually reasonable to do this based on the history, examination and a normal full blood count and ESR. In older patients, sigmoidoscopy and barium enema or colonoscopy should be performed. A plan of investigation and management should be clearly established. The symptoms tend to be persistent and are not helped by repeated normal investigations looking for an underlying cause. Symptoms may be helped by antispasmodic drugs or tricyclic antidepressants. Some patients will benefit from the consumption of a high-fibre diet.

 KEY POINTS

- Irritable bowel syndrome is a common disorder and difficult to treat.
- Explanation of the condition to the patient is an important part of the management.
- Sigmoidoscopy with air insufflation often reproduces the symptoms of IBS.

CASE 33: HEADACHES AND CONFUSION

History
A 28-year-old black South African theatre nurse in London is admitted to the emergency department complaining of headaches and confusion. Her headaches have developed over the past 3 weeks and have become progressively more severe. The headaches are now persistent and diffuse. Her friend who accompanies her says that she has lost 10 kg in weight over 6 months and has recently become increasingly confused. Her speech is slurred. While in the emergency department she has a generalized tonic–clonic convulsion.

Examination
She is thin and weighs 55 kg. Her temperature is 38.5°C. There is oral candidiasis. There is no lymphadenopathy. Examination of her cardiovascular, respiratory and gastrointestinal systems is normal. Neurological examination prior to her convulsion showed her to be disoriented in time, place and person. There were no focal neurological signs. Funduscopy shows bilateral papilloedema.

INVESTIGATIONS

		Normal
Haemoglobin	12.2 g/dL	11.7–15.7 g/dL
White cell count	12.1 × 10⁹/L	3.5–11.0 × 10⁹/L
Platelets	365 × 10⁹/L	150–440 × 10⁹/L
Sodium	126 mmol/L	135–145 mmol/L
Potassium	3.9 mmol/L	3.5–5.0 mmol/L
Urea	6.2 mmol/L	2.5–6.7 mmol/L
Creatinine	73 µmol/L	70–120 µmol/L
Glucose	5.6 mmol/L	4.0–6.0 mmol/L

A computed tomography (CT) scan is shown in Figure 33.1.

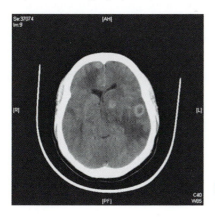

Figure 33.1 Computed tomography scan of the brain.

Questions
- What is the cause for this woman's headaches, confusion and convulsions?
- What is the underlying diagnosis?
- How should this woman be further investigated and treated?

ANSWER 33

This woman has cerebral toxoplasmosis secondary to HIV infection. This condition is caused by the protozoan *Toxoplasma gondii,* which primarily infects cats but can also be carried by any warm-blooded animal. In the West, 30–80 per cent of adults have been infected by ingesting food or water contaminated by cat faeces or by eating raw meat from sheep or pigs that contained *Toxoplasma* cysts. After ingestion by humans the organism divides rapidly within macrophages and spreads to muscles and brain. The immune system rapidly controls the infection, and the cysts remain dormant. The primary infection is generally asymptomatic but can cause an acute mononucleosis-type illness with generalized lympadenopathy and rash. It may leave scars in the choroid and retina and small inflammatory lesions in the brain. If the host then becomes immunocompromised, the organism starts proliferating, causing toxoplasmosis. This is an AIDS-defining illness but is relatively rare in solid organ transplant recipients. Cerebral toxoplasmosis usually presents with a subacute illness comprising fever; headache; confusion; convulsions; cognitive disturbance; and focal neurological signs, including hemiparesis, ataxia, cranial nerve lesions, visual field defects and sensory loss. Movement disorders are common due to involvement of the basal ganglia. CT or magnetic resonance imaging (MRI) will usually show multiple bilateral ring-enhancing lesions predominantly located near the grey–white matter junction, basal ganglia, brainstem and cerebellum. The clinical and radiological differential diagnoses include lymphoma, tuberculosis, Cryptococcus, secondary tumours and bacterial abscesses. Anti-toxoplasma IgG antibody is usually but not always positive in patients with toxoplasma encephalitis.

The other clues in this case to the diagnosis of HIV infection include the patient's country of origin, the weight loss and oral candidiasis. The headaches and papilloedema are caused by raised intracranial pressure from the multiple space-occupying lesions. The hyponatraemia is due to the syndrome of inappropriate antidiuretic hormone (ADH) secretion (SIADH) consequent to the raised intracranial pressure.

This woman should be started on anticonvulsants to prevent further seizures. Treatment is started with high-dose sulfadiazine and pyrimethamine together with folinic acid to prevent myelosuppression. There should be a rapid clinical and radiological improvement. In cases that have not responded within 3 weeks, a biopsy of one of the lesions should be considered. Cerebral toxoplamosis is uniformly fatal if untreated, and even after treatment neurological sequelae are common.

The patient should be counselled about HIV infection, and consent for an HIV test should be obtained. Her HIV viral load and CD4 count should be measured and antiretroviral drugs started. She should be advised to contact her previous sexual partners so that they can be tested and started on antiretroviral therapy. She should also tell her occupational health department so that the appropriate advice can be taken about contacting, testing and reassuring patients. The risk of HIV transmission from an HIV positive healthcare worker to a patient is very small.

 KEY POINTS

- Toxoplasmosis is the most common opportunistic infection of the central nervous system in patients with AIDS.
- Patients can present with headache, confusion, seizures and focal neurological deficits.
- The clinical and radiological response to treatment is usually rapid.

CASE 34: SEIZURES

History

A 23-year-old African-Caribbean woman is admitted to the emergency department having had two tonic–clonic generalized seizures, which were witnessed by her mother. Her mother says that her daughter has been behaving increasingly strangely and has been hearing voices talking about her. Recently, she has complained of severe headaches. She has lost weight and has noticed that her hair has been falling out. She has also complained of night sweats and flitting joint pains affecting mainly the small joints of her hands and feet. She works as a bank clerk. She smokes 5–10 cigarettes per day and consumes about 10 units of alcohol per week. She is taking no regular medication. She has no significant medical or psychiatric history.

Examination

She is drowsy but responsive to pain. There is no neck stiffness. Her scalp hair is thin and patchy. Her temperature is 38.5°C. She has numerous small palpable lymph nodes. Her pulse rate is 104/min and regular; blood pressure is 164/102 mmHg. Examination of her cardio-vascular, respiratory and abdominal systems is otherwise normal. Neurological examination reveals no focal abnormality and no papilloedema.

INVESTIGATIONS		
		Normal
Haemoglobin	7.2 g/dL	11.7–15.7 g/dL
Mean corpuscular volume (MCV)	85 fL	80–99 fL
White cell count	2.2 × 10⁹/L	3.5–11.0 × 10⁹/L
Platelets	72 × 10⁹/L	150–440 × 10⁹/L
Erythrocyte sedimentation rate (ESR)	90 mm/h	<10 mm/h
Sodium	136 mmol/L	135–145 mmol/L
Potassium	4.2 mmol/L	3.5–5.0 mmol/L
Urea	16.4 mmol/L	2.5–6.7 mmol/L
Creatinine	176 µmol/L	70–120 µmol/L
Glucose	4.8 mmol/L	4.0–6.0 mmol/L
Lumbar puncture		
Leucocytes	150/mL	<5/mL
Cerebrospinal fluid (CSF) protein	1.2 g/L	<0.4 g/L
CSF glucose	4.1 mmol/L	<70 per cent plasma glucose value

Urinalysis: +++ protein; +++ blood
Urine microscopy: ++ red cell; red cell casts present
Chest X-ray: normal
Electrocardiogram (ECG): sinus tachycardia
Computed tomography (CT) of the brain: normal
CSF Gram stain: negative

Questions
- What is the likely diagnosis?
- How would you investigate and manage this patient?

ANSWER 34

This patient has a number of important symptoms, particularly the generalized seizures, auditory hallucinations, fever, arthralgia and alopecia. Investigations show low haemoglobin, white cells and platelets with impaired renal function and blood, protein and cells in the urine. The CSF contains white cells and a high protein content but no organisms. This is a multisystem disease, and the symptoms and investigations are explained best by a diagnosis of systemic lupus erythematosus (SLE). SLE is an autoimmune condition that is about nine times more common in women than men and is especially common in African-Caribbean and Asian individuals. It varies in severity from a mild illness causing a rash or joint pains to a life-threatening multisystem illness. In the brain, SLE causes small-vessel vasculitis and can present with depression, a schizophrenia-like psychosis, seizures, chorea and focal cerebral/spinal cord infarction. MRI will show vasculitic lesions in the brain. Lumbar puncture usually shows a raised leucocyte count and protein level. Coombs-positive haemolytic anaemia may occur. Leucopenia and thrombocytopenia are common. Glomerulonephritis is another common manifestation of lupus and may present with microscopic haematuria/proteinuria, nephrotic syndrome or renal failure. Arthritis commonly affects the proximal interphalangeal and metacarpophalangeal joints and wrists, usually as arthralgia without any deformity.

> ### ❗ Differential diagnosis of the combination of headaches/psychiatric features/seizures
>
> - Meningitis/encephalitis
> - 'Recreational' drug abuse (e.g. cocaine)
> - Cerebral tumour
> - Acute alcohol withdrawal: delirium tremens
> - Hypertensive encephalopathy

This patient needs urgent antihypertensive treatment to lower her blood pressure and anticonvulsant treatment. Blood should be sent for anti-DNA antibodies (present in SLE) and complement C3 and C4 levels (depressed in SLE). A renal biopsy will provide histological evidence of the severity of the lupus nephritis. As soon as active infection has been excluded, treatment should be started with intravenous steroids and cytotoxic agents such as cyclophosphamide. Plasma exchange may be added in severe or resistant cases.

> ### 🔑 KEY POINTS
>
> - SLE is particularly common in young African-Caribbean women.
> - SLE may present with predominantly neurological or psychiatric features.
> - A low white cell count or low platelet numbers are often a suggestive feature of SLE.

CASE 35: SWELLING IN THE NECK

History
A 38-year-old man presents to his general practitioner (GP) complaining of a painless lump on the right side of his neck. This has been present for about 2 months and seems to be enlarging. He has had no recent throat infections. He has been feeling generally unwell and has lost about 5 kg in weight. The patient has also developed drenching night sweats. Simultaneously he has noticed severe generalized itching. He has had no significant past medical history. He is an accountant and is married with three children. He neither smokes nor drinks alcohol and is not taking any regular medication.

Examination
His temperature is 37.8°C. There is a smooth, firm 3 × 4 cm palpable mass in the right supraclavicular fossae. There are also lymph nodes 1–2 cm in diameter, palpable in both axillae and inguinal areas. His oropharynx appears normal. There are multiple excoriations of his skin. His pulse rate is 100/min and regular, and blood pressure is 112/66 mmHg. Examination of his cardiovascular and respiratory systems is normal. On abdominal examination, there is a mass palpable 3 cm below the left costal margin. The mass is dull to percussion, and it is impossible to palpate its upper edge. Neurological examination is normal.

🔍 INVESTIGATIONS

		Normal
Haemoglobin	11.6 g/dL	13.3–17.7 g/dL
Mean corpuscular volume (MCV)	87 fL	80–99 fL
White cell count	12.2×10^9/L	$3.9–10.6 \times 10^9$/L
Platelets	321×10^9/L	$150–440 \times 10^9$/L
Erythrocyte sedimentation rate	74 mm/h	<10 mm/h
Sodium	138 mmol/L	135–145 mmol/L
Potassium	4.2 mmol/L	3.5–5.0 mmol/L
Urea	5.2 mmol/L	2.5–6.7 mmol/L
Creatinine	114 μmol/L	70–120 μmol/L
Calcium	2.44 mmol/L	2.12–2.65 mmol/L
Phosphate	1.1 mmol/L	0.8–1.45 mmol/L
Total protein	65 g/L	60–80 g/L
Albumin	41 g/L	35–50 g/L
Bilirubin	16 mmol/L	3–17 mmol/L
Alanine transaminase	22 IU/L	5–35 IU/L
Alkaline phosphatase	228 IU/L	30–300 IU/L

Urinalysis: no protein; no blood

Questions
- What is the likely diagnosis?
- How would you investigate and manage this patient?

ANSWER 35

Transient small nodes in the neck or groin are common benign findings. However, a 3 × 4 cm mass of nodes for 2 months is undoubtedly abnormal. Persistent lymphade-nopathy and constitutional symptoms suggest a likely diagnosis of lymphoma or chronic leukaemia. Sarcoidosis and tuberculosis are possible but less likely diagnoses. Lymph nodes are normally barely palpable, if at all. The character of enlarged lymph nodes is very important. In acute infections the nodes are tender, and the overlying skin may be red. Carcinomatous nodes are usually very hard, fixed and irregular. The nodes of chronic leukaemias and lymphomas are non-tender, firm and rubbery. The distribution of enlarged lymph nodes may be diagnostic. Repeated minor trauma and infection may cause enlargement of the locally draining lymph nodes. Enlargement of the left supra-clavicular nodes may be due to metastatic spread from bronchial and nasopharyngeal carcinomas or from gastric carcinomas (Virchow's node). However, when there is gener-alized lymphadenopathy with or without splenomegaly, a systemic illness is most likely. The typical systemic symptoms of lymphoma are malaise, fever, night sweats, pruritus, weight loss, anorexia and fatigue. Fever indicates extensive disease and may be associated with night sweats. Severe skin itching is a feature of some cases of lymphoma and other myeloproliferative illnesses.

The incidence of lymphoma is greatly increased in patients who are immunosuppressed, such as organ transplant recipients and patients with HIV infection.

> **!** **Major differential diagnosis of generalized lymphadenopathy**
>
> - *Infections*: infectious mononucleosis or 'glandular fever' (caused by Epstein–Barr virus infection), toxoplasmosis, cytomegalovirus infection, acute HIV infection, tuberculosis, brucellosis and syphilis.
> - *Inflammatory conditions*: systemic lupus erythematosus, rheumatoid arthritis and sarcoidosis.
> - *Lymphomas or chronic lymphocytic leukaemia.*

The most likely clinical diagnosis in this man is lymphoma. The patient should be referred to a local haemato-oncology unit. He should have a lymph node biopsy to reach a histological diagnosis and a computed tomography (CT) scan of the thorax, abdomen and bone mar-row to stage the disease. CT scanning is a non-invasive and effective method of imaging retroperitoneal, iliac and mesenteric nodes. Positron emission tomography (PET) combined with CT increases the sensitivity for detecting disease (Figure 35.1) and is useful for assess-ing response to treatment. The patient will require treatment with radiotherapy and chemo-therapy. Radiotherapy alone is reserved for patients with limited disease, but this patient has widespread disease. He should be given allopurinol prior to starting chemotherapy to prevent massive release of uric acid as a consequence of tumour lysis, which can cause acute renal failure.

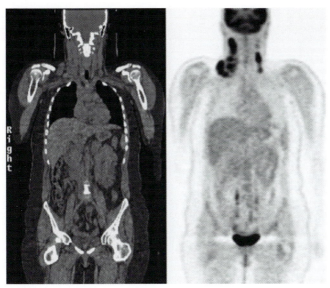

Figure 35.1 CT–PET image showing increased activity in enlarged lymph nodes, particularly in the right side of the neck.

🔑 **KEY POINTS**

- The character and distribution of abnormal lymph nodes is helpful in reaching a diagnosis.
- Lymphadenopathy affecting two or more separate groups of nodes suggests lymphoma or a systemic infection.
- CT–PET scanning allows accurate staging of disease and assessment of maintenance of remission in response to treatment.

CASE 36: ABDOMINAL PAIN

History

A 74-year-old woman has a 10-year history of intermittent lower abdominal pain. The pain has been colicky in nature and is associated with a feeling of distension in the left iliac fossa. It is generally relieved by passing flatus or faeces. She tends to be constipated and passes small pieces of faeces. Four years previously she passed some blood with her bowel motion and had a barium enema performed. The X-ray of this is shown in Figure 36.1. Over the last week her pain has worsened, and now she has continuous pain in the left iliac fossa and feels generally unwell. Her appetite has been poor over this same time. She has not had her bowels open over the last 2 days. In her previous medical history she had a hysterectomy for fibroids 20 years ago. There is a family history of ischaemic heart disease and diabetes mellitus. She lives alone and does her own cooking and shopping.

Examination

She has a temperature of 38.5°C, and her abdomen is tender with a vague impression of a mass in the left iliac fossa. There is no guarding or rebound tenderness, and the bowel sounds are normal. Her pulse is 84/min, and blood pressure is 154/88 mmHg. No abnormalities are found in the respiratory system.

INVESTIGATIONS		
		Normal
Haemoglobin	11.8 g/dL	11.7–15.7 g/dL
Mean corpuscular volume (MCV)	85 fL	80–99 fL
White cell count	15.6 × 10⁹/L	3.5–11.0 × 10⁹/L
Platelets	235 × 10⁹/L	150–440 × 10⁹/L
C-reactive protein (CRP)	56 mg/L	<5 mg/L

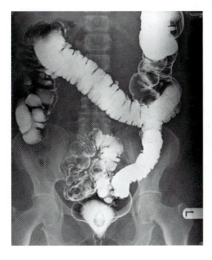

Figure 36.1 Barium enema.

Questions
- What is the likely diagnosis?
- What should be the initial management?

ANSWER 36

This woman has diverticulitis. Colonic diverticula are small outpouchings that are most commonly found in the left colon. They are very common in the elderly Western population, probably due to a deficiency in dietary fibre. Symptomatic diverticular disease has many of the features of irritable bowel syndrome. Inflammation in a diverticulum is termed diverticulitis. In severe cases, perforation, paracolic abscess formation or septicaemia may develop. Other potential complications include bowel obstruction, formation of a fistula into the rectum or vagina, and haemorrhage.

The barium enema from 4 years ago shows evidence of diverticular disease with outpouchings of the mucosa in the sigmoid colon. This would be consistent with the long-standing history of abdominal pain of colonic type and tendency to constipation. The recent problems with increased pain, tenderness, fever, raised white cell count and CRP and a mass in the left iliac fossa would be compatible with an acute exacerbation of her diverticular disease. In her case there is no evidence of peritonitis, which would signal a possible perforation of one of the diverticula.

The differential diagnosis, with the suggestion of a mass and change in bowel habit, would be carcinoma of the colon or Crohn's disease. In the absence of evidence of perforation with leak of bowel contents into the peritoneum (no peritonitis) or obstruction (normal bowel sounds, no general distension), treatment should be based on the presumptive diagnosis of diverticulitis. A colonoscopy should be performed at a later date to exclude the possibility of a colonic neoplasm.

A computed tomography (CT) scan of the abdomen will delineate the mass and suggest whether there is evidence of local abscess or fistula formation. Treatment should include broad-spectrum antibiotics (ciprofloxacin and metroridazole), intravenous fluids and rest. Further investigations are indicated, including urea and electrolytes, creatinine, glucose values; liver function tests; and blood cultures. A colonoscopy should be performed at a later date to exclude the possibility of a colonic neoplasm.

Repeated severe episodes, bleeding or obstruction may necessitate surgery. Patients are advised to eat a high fibre diet once the acute episode has subsided.

 KEY POINTS

- Diverticular disease is a common finding in the elderly Western population and may be asymptomatic or cause irritable bowel syndrome-type symptoms.
- Diverticular disease is a common condition; its presence can distract the unwary doctor from pursuing a coincident condition.
- Diverticulitis needs to be treated with antibiotics to reduce the chance of complications occurring, such as perforation or fistula formation.

CASE 37: HIGH BLOOD PRESSURE

History

A 36-year-old woman is referred by her general practitioner (GP) to a hypertension clinic. She was noted to be hypertensive when she joined the practice 2 years previously. Her blood pressure has been difficult to control, and she is currently taking four agents (bendroflumethiazide, atenolol, amlodipine and doxazosin). She had normal blood pressure and no pre-eclampsia during her only pregnancy 9 years previously. There is no family history of premature hypertension. She smokes 20 cigarettes a day and drinks less than 10 units a week. She is not on an oral contraceptive pill. She works part-time as a teaching assistant.

Examination

She is not overweight and looks well. Her pulse rate is 68/min and blood pressure is 180/102 mmHg. There is no radiofemoral delay. There are no café-au-lait spots or neurofibromas. Examination of the cardiovascular, respiratory and abdominal systems is normal. The fundi show no significant changes of hypertension.

INVESTIGATIONS		
		Normal
Haemoglobin	13.3 g/dL	11.7–15.7 g/dL
White cell count	6.2×10^9/L	$3.5–11.0 \times 10^9$/L
Platelets	266×10^9/L	$150–440 \times 10^9$/L
Sodium	139 mmol/L	135–145 mmol/L
Potassium	4.4 mmol/L	3.5–5.0 mmol/L
Urea	10.7 mmol/L	2.5–6.7 mmol/L
Creatinine	136 µmol/L	70–120 µmol/L
Albumin	42 g/L	35–50 g/L

Urinalysis: no protein; no blood
Renal ultrasound: normal-size kidneys

Results of a renal angiogram are shown in Figure 37.1.

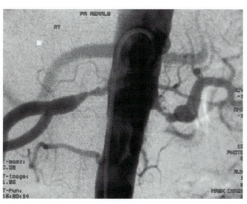

Figure 37.1 Renal angiogram.

Questions

- What is the diagnosis?
- How would be the appropriate management of this patient?

ANSWER 37

This woman has hypertension due to renovascular disease. The great majority of cases of hypertension are due to essential hypertension. Risk factors for essential hypertension include a family history of hypertension, obesity and lack of exercise. She does not have paroxysmal symptoms of sweating, palpitations and anxiety to suggest a phaeochromocytoma. There are no clinical features to suggest coarctation of the aorta (radiofemoral delay) or neurofibromatosis (café-au-lait spots/neurofibromas). Serum potassium is not low even on thiazide treatment, making Conn's syndrome or Cushing's syndrome unlikely. The principal abnormality is the modestly raised creatinine, suggesting mildly impaired renal function. The absence of haematuria and proteinuria excludes glomerulonephritis. Therefore renovascular disease needs to be considered. The absence of a renal bruit on auscultation of the abdomen does not exclude the possibility of renovascular disease. The renal angiogram shows bilateral fibromuscular dysplasia (FMD).

The commonest cause of renovascular disease is atherosclerotic renal artery stenosis (ARAS). This is common in elderly patients with evidence of generalized atherosclerosis (peripheral vascular disease and coronary artery disease). Ultrasound will often show small kidneys, and renal impairment is common. ARAS is a common cause of end-stage renal failure in the elderly.

At this woman's age atherosclerotic renovascular disease is very unlikely. FMD is the second commonest cause of renovascular disease. The commonest form is medial fibroplasia, with thinning of the intima and media leading to formation of aneurysms alternating with stenoses, presenting the classic 'string-of-beads' appearance on angiography. It predominantly affects young and middle-aged women, with a peak incidence in the fourth decade of life. Cigarette smoking is a risk factor. FMD usually presents with hypertension but can rarely present with 'flash' pulmonary oedema. FMD can also affect the carotid arteries, causing a variety of neurological symptoms.

Treatment is with percutaneous transluminal renal angioplasty. Unlike atheromatous renovascular disease, the hypertension in FMD cases is often cured, leading to complete cessation of blood pressure medication. Restenosis is rare.

 KEY POINTS

- FMD is an important cause of hypertension in young and middle-aged women.
- Renal artery angioplasty will improve or even cure hypertension in many patients with FMD.
- FMD is a very rare cause of end-stage renal failure.

CASE 38: SWELLING ON THE LEGS

History

A 34-year-old woman presents to her general practitioner (GP) complaining of a rash. Over the past 2 weeks she has developed multiple tender red swellings on her shins and forearms. The older swellings are darker in colour and seem to be healing from the centre. She feels generally unwell and tired and has pains in her wrists and ankles. She has not had a recent sore throat. Over the past 2 years she has had recurrent aphthous ulcers in her mouth. She has had no genital ulceration, but she has been troubled by intermittent abdominal pain and diarrhoea. She works as a waitress and is unmarried. She smokes about 15 cigarettes per day and drinks alcohol only occasionally. She has had no other previous medical illnesses, and there is no relevant family history that she can recall.

Examination

She is thin but looks well. There are no aphthous ulcers to see at the time of the examination. Her joints are not inflamed, and the range of movement is not restricted or painful. Examining the skin, there are multiple tender lesions on the shins and forearms. The lesions are raised and vary from 1 to 3 cm in diameter. The fresher lesions are red, and the older ones look like bruises. Physical examination is otherwise normal.

🔍 INVESTIGATIONS

		Normal
Haemoglobin	13.5 g/dL	11.7–15.7 g/dL
White cell count	15.4 × 10⁹/L	3.5–11.0 × 10⁹/L
Platelets	198 × 10⁹/L	150–440 × 10⁹/L
Erythrocyte sedimentation rate (ESR)	98 mm/h	<10 mm/h
Sodium	138 mmol/L	135–145 mmol/L
Potassium	4.3 mmol/L	3.5–5.0 mmol/L
Urea	5.4 mmol/L	2.5–6.7 mmol/L
Creatinine	86 μmol/L	70–120 μmol/L
Glucose	5.8 mmol/L	4.0–6.0 mmol/L

Chest X-ray: normal
Urinalysis: normal

Questions

- What is the diagnosis?
- What are the major causes of this condition?

ANSWER 38

This patient has erythema nodosum, in this case secondary to previously undiagnosed Crohn's disease. Erythema nodosum is due to inflammation of the small blood vessels in the deep dermis. Characteristically it affects the shins, but it may also affect the thighs and fore-arms. The number and size of the lesions are variable. Lesions tend to heal from the centre and spread peripherally. The rash is often preceded by systemic symptoms—fever, malaise and arthralgia. It usually resolves over 3–4 weeks, but persistence or recurrence suggests an underlying disease.

 Diseases linked to erythema nodosum

Streptococcal infection	Lymphoma/leukaemia
Tuberculosis	Sarcoidosis
Leprosy	Pregnancy/oral contraceptive
Glandular fever	Reaction to sulphonamides
Histoplasmosis	Ulcerative colitis
Coccidioidomycosis	Crohn's disease

The history of mouth ulcers, abdominal pain and diarrhoea strongly suggests that this woman has Crohn's disease. She should therefore be referred to a gastroenterologist for investigations, which should include a small-bowel enema and colonoscopy with biopsies. Treatment of her underlying disease with steroids should cause the erythema nodosum to resolve. With no serious underlying condition, erythema nodosum usually settles with non-steroidal anti-inflammatory drugs.

KEY POINTS

- Patients presenting with erythema nodosum should be investigated for an underlying disease.
- Erythema nodosum is most often seen on the shins but can affect the extensor surface of the forearms or thighs.

CASE 39: SHORTNESS OF BREATH AND REDUCED URINE OUTPUT

History

A 73-year-old woman presents to the emergency department complaining of increasing breathlessness over the previous 4 days. She had felt unwell for 2 months and has lost 4 kg in weight. She has had frequent nosebleeds, and over the past few days has coughed up small amounts of fresh blood. She notices that she has been passing less urine in the past few days. She has no significant past medical history.

Examination

On examination, she is febrile (38 °C), centrally cyanosed and looks unwell. She has a purpuric rash over her ankles. Her pulse is 104/min, blood pressure 160/100 mmHg. Her jugular venous pressure is not raised. Her heart sounds are normal with no added sounds. Her respiratory rate is 30 breaths/min, expansion is reduced, percussion and tactile vocal fremitus are normal but she has coarse inspiratory crackles throughout both lung fields. Her abdominal and neurological examination is normal.

🔍 INVESTIGATIONS

		Normal
Haemoglobin	10.1 g/dL	11.7–15.7 g/dL
Mean corpuscular volume (MCV)	87 fL	80–99 fL
White cell count	17.2×10^9/L	$3.9–11.0 \times 10^9$/L
Platelets	540×10^9/L	$150–440 \times 10^9$/L
Sodium	137 mmol/L	135–145 mmol/L
Potassium	6.6 mmol/L	3.5–5.0 mmol/L
Urea	45.1 mmol/L	2.5–6.7 mmol/L
Creatinine	832 µmol/L	70–120 µmol/L
Albumin	32 g/L	35–50 g/L
Calcium	2.23 mmol/L	2.12–2.65 mmol/L
Phosphate	1.9 mmol/L	0.8–1.4 mmol/L
CRP	323 mg/L	<5 mg/L
Arterial blood gases on air:		
pH	7.18	7.38–7.44
pCO_2	5.1 kPa	4.7–6.0 kPa
pO_2	6.4 kPa	12.0–14.5 kPa
Urinalysis	++ protein	+++ blood

Electrocardiogram (ECG): sinus tachycardia
Chest X-ray: Figure 39.1

Questions
- What is the likely diagnosis?
- How would you manage and investigate this patient?

ANSWER 39

This patient has respiratory and renal failure. Respiratory failure may occur due to fluid over-load in renal failure but the findings on examination (normal jugular venous pressure, coarse pan-inspiratory crackles rather than fine, late inspiratory crackles) do not support this. The chest X-ray shows bilateral infiltrates. The purpuric rash and the raised platelet count and CRP are typical of active vasculitis. Alveolar haemorrhage may produce hypoxia and radio-graphic shadowing without gross haemoptysis.

Major causes of pulmonary/renal syndrome are

- *Systemic vasculitis*: granulomatosis with polyangiitis (GPA) or Wegner's is a vascu-litis of the medium and small arteries producing a granulomatous inflammation of the upper and lower respiratory tracts and a necrotizing glomerulonephritis. Microscopic polyarteritis primarily affects the venules, capillaries and arterioles and can cause pulmonary haemorrhage and a similar renal lesion. Patients with both diseases usually have antineutrophilic cytoplasmic antibodies (ANCA).
- *Antiglomerular basement membrane disease*: Goodpasture's disease.
- *Systemic lupus erythematosus.*

The history of nosebleeds implying upper respiratory tract involvement suggests that the most likely diagnosis is GPA granulomatosis with polyangiitis (Wegener's) rather than microscopic polyarteritis. Both are conditions of small vessel vasculitis and cause necrotiz-ing glomerulonephritis and pulmonary haemorrhage, and can affect other organs such as the skin, joints, eyes and nervous system. Antiglomerular basement membrane disease does not cause a rash. The other principal differential diagnoses of vasculitis include atheroembolic disease, infective endocarditis and meningococcal septicaemia.

This woman needs emergency treatment for her respiratory failure, metabolic acidosis and hyperkalaemia. She requires oxygen and may require non-invasive or mechanical ventila-tion. Her hyperkalaemia needs emergency treatment with intravenous calcium gluconate and an infusion of dextrose and insulin until dialysis or haemofiltration is being organised.

All patients with acute renal failure should have a renal ultrasound to size the kidneys and rule out obstruction. A renal biopsy in this patient will provide histological confirmation of systemic vasculitis by showing a focal necrotizing glomerulonephritis usually with crescent formation. Biopsy of nasal lesions is often unproductive, showing only necrotic tissue and may delay diagnosis. Blood should be sent for ANCA which are present in about 90% of untreated cases of small vessel vasculitis. Her gas transfer factor will be temporarily increased because of her pulmonary haemorrhage.

The specific treatment for this woman is urgent plasma exchange and immunosuppression with steroids and cyclophosphamide. After the acute phase, maintenance treatment is with prednisolone and azathioprine. Rituximab is increasingly used as an alternative to cyclo-phosphamide especially in cases of relapsing vasculitis.

 KEY POINTS

- Clinical symptoms of GPA affecting the lungs are cough, breathlessness and haemoptysis.
- ANCA is present in over 90% of cases of GPA causing pulmonary/renal involvement.
- Rapid treatment is essential to prevent irreversible tissue necrosis.

CASE 40: PAIN IN THE CHEST AND SHORTNESS OF BREATH

History
A 17-year-old African-Caribbean boy presents to the emergency department complaining of severe chest pain and shortness of breath. He has had a sore throat for a few days and started developing pain in his back and arms, which has increased in severity. Six hours prior to admission he suddenly developed right-sided chest pain, which is worse on inspiration and associated with marked breathlessness. He has had previous episodes of pains affecting his fingers and back, for which he has taken codeine and ibuprofen. He was born in London and lives with his parents and younger sister. He is attending school and has had no problems there. There is no family history of note.

Examination
He is unwell, febrile (37.8°C) and cyanosed. His conjunctivae are pale. Pulse rate is 112/min and regular, and blood pressure is 136/85 mmHg. His jugular venous pressure is not raised, and heart sounds are normal. His respiratory rate is 28/min, and a right pleural rub is audible. Abdominal and neurological examination is normal. There are no rashes on the skin and no joint abnormalities.

🔍 INVESTIGATIONS

		Normal
Haemoglobin	7.6 g/dL	13.3–17.7 g/dL
Mean corpuscular volume (MCV)	86 fL	80–99 fL
White cell count	16 × 10⁹/L	3.9–10.6 × 10⁹/L
Platelets	162 × 10⁹/L	150–440 × 10⁹/L
Sodium	139 mmol/L	135–145 mmol/L
Potassium	4.4 mmol/L	3.5–5.0 mmol/L
Urea	6.2 mmol/L	2.5–6.7 mmol/L
Creatinine	94 µmol/L	70–120 µmol/L
Bicarbonate	24 mmol/L	24–30 mmol/L
Arterial blood gases on air:		
pH	7.33	7.38–7.44
pCO_2	2.6 kPa	4.7–6.0 kPa
pO_2	7.2 kPa	12.0–14.5 kPa

Electrocardiogram (ECG): sinus tachycardia
Chest X-ray: normal

Questions
- What is the likely diagnosis?
- How would you investigate and manage this patient?

ANSWER 40

This boy has sickle cell disease and presents with his first serious bony/chest crisis. Sickle cell disease occurs mainly in African black populations and sporadically in the Mediterranean and Middle East. Haemoglobin S differs from haemoglobin A by the substitution of valine for glutamic acid at position 6 in the b-chain. Sickled cells have increased mechanical fragility and a shortened survival, leading to haemolytic anaemia, and can block small vessels, leading to tissue infarction. Sickle cell disease has a very variable clinical course due to a combination of reasons, including the haemoglobin F (HbF) level and socioeconomic factors. It usually presents in early childhood with anaemia and jaundice due to chronic haemolytic anaemia or painful hands and feet with inflammation of the fingers due to dactylitis. This patient is having a pulmonary crisis characterized by pleuritic chest pain, shortness of breath and hypoxia. It is usually precipitated by dehydration or infection (in this case, a sore throat). The principal differential diagnoses of a patient presenting with pleuritic pain and breathlessness are pneumonia, pneumothorax and pulmonary emboli.

> **! Major potential complications of sickle cell disease**
>
> - Thrombotic: causes generalized or localized bony pains, abdominal crises, chest crises, neurological signs or priapism.
> - Aplastic crises: triggered by parvovirus infection.
> - Haemolytic anaemia.
> - Sequestration crises in children with rapid enlargement of the liver and spleen, usually in young children.
> - Aseptic necrosis: often of the humeral or femoral heads.
> - Renal failure due to renal medullary infarction or glomerular disease. Hyposplenism due to autoinfarction in childhood.

This patient should be admitted for rest, intravenous fluids, oxygen and adequate analgesia. He has a low arterial pO_2 and appears cyanosed. Cyanosis is more difficult to detect in the presence of anaemia. Infection should be treated with antibiotics. A blood film will show sickled erythrocytes and elevated reticulocyte count. The definitive investigation is haemoglobin electrophoresis, which will demonstrate HbS, absent HbA and a variable HbF level. Partial exchange transfusion may be needed to reduce the level of his sickle cells to less than 30 per cent. He should be followed up by an expert sickle team since this has been shown to reduce admissions and improve quality of care. He may benefit from long-term hydroxyurea, which raises the HbF level and reduces the number of crises.

> ** KEY POINTS**
>
> - In African-Caribbean patients, sickle cell disease should be thought of as a cause of chest or abdominal pain.
> - Patients with sickle cell disease should be looked after in specialized haematology units with psychological support available.
> - Severe thrombotic complications should be treated with partial exchange transfusion.

CASE 41: ABDOMINAL PAIN

History

A 44-year-old woman presents to her general practitioner (GP) complaining of pain in her epigastrium radiating into her back. The pain developed 18 hours earlier and has become progressively more severe. She has not eaten for the last 24 hours and has vomited altered food and then fluid but no blood on 4 occasions. She has had some looseness of her bowel motions.

She feels feverish and increasingly unwell. She has no pain on passing urine and no urinary frequency. Her last menstrual period was 2 weeks ago.

She had similar but much milder pains lasting 2–3 days 3–4 months ago. She has no other significant past medical history.

She smokes 15–20 cigarettes per day, drinks around half a bottle of wine each night. She has not used any recreational drugs.

Examination

She looks unwell. Her temperature is 38.8°C. Her pulse rate is 110/min, and blood pressure 102/64 mmHg. In the respiratory system there is some dullness to percussion at the left base. She is tender to palpation in the epigastrium and the centre of the abdomen. There is some guarding, and rebound tenderness around the umbilicus. There is a suggestion of some skin discolouration in the flanks. Bowel sounds are sparse. Rectal examination is normal; there is some brown poorly formed stool on the examination glove.

INVESTIGATIONS		
		Normal
Haemoglobin	15.3 g/dL	11.7–15.7 g/dL
White cell count	15.2 × 10⁹/L	3.5–11.0 × 10⁹/L
Platelets	412 × 10⁹/L	150–440 × 10⁹/L
Sodium	140 mmol/L	135–145 mmol/L
Potassium	3.5 mmol/L	3.5–5.0 mmol/L
Urea	9.3 mmol/L	2.5–6.7 mmol/L
Creatinine	82 μmol/L	70–120 μmol/L
C-reactive protein (CRP)	192 mg/L	<5 mg/L

Urinalysis: trace protein; trace blood; nitrites negative
Chest X-ray: small left-side pleural effusion
Abdominal X-ray: normal

Questions
- What is the diagnosis?
- How would you assess and manage this patient?

ANSWER 41

The most likely diagnosis is acute pancreatitis. This most commonly presents with central or epigastric pain which radiates to the back. A posteriorly perforating duodenal ulcer may produce a similar pattern of pain. Nausea, vomiting and fever are common and fluid loss leads to haemodynamic instability and shock. The tachycardia, low blood pressure and haemoconcentration suggest fluid depletion. On examination there are signs of peritonitis. In severe cases of acute pancreatitis haemorrhage may produce blood staining in the skin of the flanks (Grey–Turner's sign) or around the umbilicus (Cullen's sign). Pleural effusions may occur especially on the left, or pulmonary oedema. The raised white count and high CRP reflect the associated severe inflammation in acute pancreatitis.

The most common precipitating causes of acute pancreatitis are excessive alcohol use and gallstones together, which account for 75% of cases. Other less common causes are hypercalcaemia, hyperlipidaemia, abdominal trauma, drugs such as corticosteroids, diuretics, pentamidine, azathioprine, infections such as mumps, coxsackie virus and cytalomegalovirus.

Diagnosis is based on the clinical picture and raised levels of serum amylase or lipase. Elevations of amylase can occur also in mesenteric ischaemia and other acute abdominal conditions but an amylase more than 3 times the upper limit of normal with typical clinical features is diagnostic. Imaging such as CT scan can show inflammation in the pancreas but is not usually necessary. Ultrasound may show underlying biliary tract disease but is less sensitive in the setting of acute pancreatitis. Magnetic resonance cholangiopancreatography (MRCP) can also be used in the diagnosis of suspected biliary and pancreatic duct obstruction.

Various staging criteria have been used to grade the severity of acute pancreatitis. The Ransom criteria are widely used for alcohol induced disease, applied up to 48 hours after onset:

on admission:

- > 55 years
- WBC count >16 × 10^9/L
- Blood glucose >10mmol/L
- Serum LDH >350 IU/L
- AST level >250 IU/L

up to 48 hours:

- Hematocrit fall >10%
- Urea increased >1.8 mmol/L
- Serum calcium <2.0 mmol/L
- P_aO_2 <8.0 kPa
- Base deficit >4 mEq/L
- Estimated fluid sequestration >600 mL

With one point for each item, a score of >2 is predictive of severe pancreatitis and warrants admission to the intensive care unit. Alternative scores such as the Glasgow criteria are often used.

Management is largely related to fluid replacement and analgesia while keeping the patient nil by mouth. There is often considerable fluid loss retro- and intraperitoneally. Antibiotic treatment is still uncertain and is not generally used routinely.

Systemic complications may be related to inflammation and fluid loss, acute respiratory distress syndrome, multiple organ dysfunction, or pancreatic damage producing diabetes.

Hypocalcameia may occur as calcium is involved in saponification (soap formation) of fats retroperitoneally. Local complications are related to pancreatic necrosis, secondary infection and development of pancreatic pseudocysts.

 Differential diagnosis of acute pancreatitis

Other conditions to consider are

- Pancreatic pseudocyst
- Pancreatic dysfunction (diabetes mellitus; malabsorption due to exocrine failure)
- Pancreatic cancer

Although these are common symptoms, they are not always present. Simple abdominal pain may be the sole symptom. The most common causes are

- Alcohol
- Gallstones
- Metabolic disorders: hereditary pancreatitis, hypercalcemia, hyperlipidemia, malnutrition
- Abdominal trauma
- Penetrating ulcers
- Malignancy
- Drugs: steroids, sulfonamides, furosemide, thiazides
- Infections: mumps, coxsackie virus, mycoplasma pneumoniae, ascaris, clonorchis
- Structural abnormalities: choledochocele, pancreas divisum.

KEY POINTS

- The common causes of acute pancreatitis are alcohol and gallstone disease.
- The diagnosis of acute pancreatitis relies on the clinical picture and serum amylase or lipase.
- Adequate fluid replacement is an important part of management.

CASE 42: POSTOPERATIVE DETERIORATION

History
The medical team is asked to review a postoperative surgical patient. A 62-year-old lady had been admitted 10 days previously to have a right hemicolectomy performed for a caecal carcinoma. This was discovered on colonoscopy, which was performed to investigate iron-deficiency anaemia and change in bowel habit. She is otherwise fit with no significant medical history. She is a retired teacher. She neither smokes nor drinks alcohol and is on no medication. Her preoperative serum creatinine was 76 μmol/L. The initial surgery was uneventful, and she was given cefuroxime and metronidazole as routine antibiotic prophylaxis. However, the patient developed a prolonged ileus associated with abdominal pain. On postoperative day 5, the patient started to spike fevers up to 38.5°C and was commenced on intravenous gentamicin 80 mg 8 hourly in addition to the other antibiotics. Over the next 5 days she remained persistently febrile, with negative blood cultures. In the last 24 h, she has also become relatively hypotensive, with her systolic blood pressure around 95 mmHg despite intravenous colloids. Her urine output is now 15 mL/h.

Examination
She is unwell and sweating profusely. She is jaundiced. Her pulse rate is 110/min regular, blood pressure is 95/60 mmHg, and jugular venous pressure is not raised. Her heart sounds are normal. Her respiratory rate is 30/min. Her breath sounds are normal. Her abdomen is tender, with guarding over the right iliac fossa. Bowel sounds are absent.

🔍 INVESTIGATIONS

		Normal
Haemoglobin	8.2 g/dL	11.7–15.7 g/dL
Mean corpuscular volume (MCV)	83 fL	80–99 fL
White cell count	26.3 × 10⁹/L	3.5–11.0 × 10⁹/L
Platelets	94 × 10⁹/L	150–440 × 10⁹/L
Sodium	126 mmol/L	135–145 mmol/L
Potassium	5.8 mmol/L	3.5–5.0 mmol/L
Bicarbonate	6 mmol/L	24–30 mmol/L
Urea	36.2 mmol/L	2.5–6.7 mmol/L
Creatinine	523 μmol/L	70–120 μmol/L
Glucose	2.6 mmol/L	4.0–6.0 mmol/L
Albumin	31 g/L	35–50 g/L
Bilirubin	95 mmol/L	3–17 mmol/L
Alanine transaminase	63 IU/L	5–35 IU/L
Alkaline phosphatase	363 IU/L	30–300 IU/L
Trough gentamicin level	4.8 mg/mL	<2.0 mg/mL

Urinalysis: + blood; + protein; granular casts and epithelial cells

Questions
- What are the causes of this patient's acute renal failure?
- How would you further investigate and manage this patient?

ANSWER 42

This woman has postoperative acute renal failure due to a combination of intra-abdominal sepsis and aminoglycoside nephrotoxicity. Her sepsis is due to an anastomotic leak with localized peritonitis, which has been partially controlled with antibiotics. Her sepsis syndrome is manifested by fever, tachycardia, hypotension, hypoglycaemia, metabolic acidosis (low bicarbonate) and oliguria. The low sodium and high potassium are common in this condition as cell membrane function becomes less effective. The elevated white count is a marker for bacterial infection, and the low platelet count is part of the picture of disseminated intravascular coagulation. Jaundice and abnormal liver function tests are common features of intra-abdominal sepsis. Aminoglycosides (gentamicin, streptomycin, amikacin) cause auditory and vestibular dysfunction, as well as acute renal failure. Risk factors for aminoglycoside nephrotoxicity are higher doses and duration of treatment, increased age, pre-existing renal insufficiency, hepatic failure and volume depletion. Aminoglycoside nephrotoxicity usually occurs 7–10 days after starting treatment. Monitoring of trough levels is important, although an increase in the trough level generally indicates decreased excretion of the drug caused by a fall in the glomerular flow rate. Thus, nephrotoxicity may be already established by the time the trough level rises.

This patient needs urgent resuscitation. She requires transfer to the intensive care unit, where she will need invasive circulatory monitoring with an arterial line and central venous pressure line to allow accurate assessment of her colloid and inotrope requirements. She also needs urgent renal replacement therapy to correct her acidosis and hyperkalaemia. In a haemodynamically unstable patient like this, continuous haemofiltration is the preferred method. She also needs urgent surgical review. The abdomen should be imaged with either ultrasound or computed tomography (CT) scanning to try to identify any collection of pus. Once haemodynamically stable, the patient should have a laparotomy to drain any collection and form a temporary colostomy.

 KEY POINTS

- Postoperative acute renal failure is often multifactorial due to hypotension, sepsis and the use of nephrotoxic drugs such as aminoglycosides and non-steroidal anti-inflammatory drugs (NSAIDs).
- Aminoglycoside drugs are extremely valuable for treating Gram-negative infections, but levels must be monitored to avoid toxicity.
- Sepsis syndrome must be recognized early and treated aggressively to reduce the morbidity and mortality of this condition.

CASE 43: ABDOMINAL DISCOMFORT

History

A 64-year-old woman with a 6-month history of mild abdominal discomfort is referred to out-patients. This discomfort has been intermittent and involved the right iliac fossa mainly. There has been no particular relation to eating or to bowel movements. Over this time her appetite has gone down a little, and she thinks that she has lost around 5 kg in weight. The intensity of the pain has become slightly worse over this time, and it is now present on most days.

Over the last 6 weeks she has developed some new symptoms. She has developed a different sort of cramping abdominal pain located mainly in the right iliac fossa. This pain has been associated with a feeling of the need to pass her motions and often with some diarrhoea. During these episodes her husband has commented that she looked red in the face, but she has associated this with the abdominal discomfort and the embarrassment from the urgent need to have her bowels open.

There is no other relevant previous medical history. She has smoked 15 cigarettes daily for the last 45 years, and she drinks around 7 units of alcohol each week. She has noticed a little breathlessness on occasions over the last few months and has heard herself wheeze on several occasions. She has never had any problems with asthma, and there is no family history of asthma or other atopic conditions.

She worked as a school secretary for 30 years and has never had a job involving any industrial exposure. She has no pets. She has lived all her life in London, and her only trip outside the UK was a day trip to France.

🔍 INVESTIGATIONS

A computed tomography (CT) scan of her abdomen was performed and is shown in Figure 43.1.

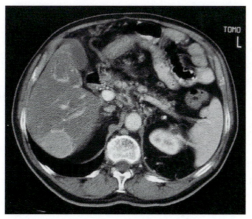

Figure 43.1 Computed tomography scan of the abdomen.

Questions

- What diagnoses should be considered?
- What investigations should be performed?

ANSWER 43

The symptoms she describes raise the possibility of a 5-hydroxytryptamine (5-HT)-secreting carcinoid tumour. The typical clinical features of the carcinoid syndrome are facial flushing, abdominal cramps and diarrhoea. Sometimes there is asthma and right-sided heart valve problems. The symptoms are characteristically intermittent and may come at times of increased release on activity. Skin changes may be persistent.

The CT scan of the liver shows a space-occupying lesion in the liver likely to represent a metastasis to the liver. Fluid-containing cystic lesions are of lower density. Other secondary tumours would give a similar appearance. Carcinoids do not generally produce their symptoms until they have metastasized to the liver from their original site, which is usually in the small bowel. In the small bowel the tumours may produce local symptoms of obstruction or bleeding.

The symptoms of carcinoid tumours are related to the secretion of 5-HT by the tumour. The diagnosis depends on finding a high level of the metabolite 5-hydroxyindole acetic acid (5-HIAA) in a 24-h collection of urine. Histology can be obtained from a liver biopsy guided to the correct area by ultrasound or CT.

The symptoms can be controlled by antagonists of 5-HT, such as cyproheptadine, or by inhibitors of its synthesis (p-chlorophenylalanine) or release (octreotide). The tumour can be reduced in size with consequent lessening of symptoms by embolization of its arterial supply using interventional radiology techniques.

When odd symptoms such as those described here occur, the diagnosis of carcinoid tumour should always be remembered and investigated. In real life, most of the investigations for suspected carcinoid turn out to be negative.

Carcinoid tumours can occur in the lung where they act as slowly growing malignant tumours. From the lung they can eventually be associated with left heart-valve problems. The other typical carcinoid features occur only after metastasis to the liver.

 KEY POINTS

- Intermittent skin flushing, diarrhoea, wheezing and abdominal cramps are symptoms of the carcinoid syndrome.
- All these symptoms have much commoner causes.
- Metastasis to the liver is present before the symptoms of carcinoid syndrome occur.

CASE 44: UNCONSCIOUS AT HOME

History

A 28-year-old woman is admitted to the emergency department in a coma. The patient was found unconscious on the floor by her boyfriend. She had not been seen by anyone for the previous 48 hours. No history was available from the patient, but her partner volunteered the information that they are both intravenous heroin addicts. She is unemployed, smokes 25 cigarettes per day, drinks 40 units of alcohol per week and has used heroin for the past 4 years. They have occasionally shared needles with other addicts. They both had negative HIV tests about 1 year ago. She has not made any suicide attempts in the past. She has had no other medical illnesses. She has lost touch with her family.

Examination

There are multiple old scarred needle puncture sites. Her pulse is 64/min and regular, blood pressure is 110/60 mmHg, jugular venous pressure is not raised, and heart sounds are normal. Her respiratory rate is 12/min, and she has dullness to percussion and bronchial breathing at the left base posteriorly. Abdominal examination is normal. Her consciousness level is depressed, but she is rousable to painful stimuli. She has pinpoint pupils but has no focal neurological signs. A bolus injection of intravenous naloxone causes her conscious level to rise transiently. Her left arm is swollen and painful from the shoulder down.

INVESTIGATIONS

		Normal
Haemoglobin	13.6 g/dL	13.3–17.7 g/dL
White cell count	9.2 × 10⁹/L	3.9–10.6 × 10⁹/L
Platelets	233 × 10⁹/L	150–440 × 10⁹/L
Sodium	137 mmol/L	135–145 mmol/L
Potassium	7.8 mmol/L	3.5–5.0 mmol/L
Urea	42.3 mmol/L	2.5–6.7 mmol/L
Creatinine	622 µmol/L	70–120 µmol/L
Bicarbonate	14 mmol/L	24–30 mmol/L
Glucose	4.1 mmol/L	4.0–6.0 mmol/L
Calcium	1.64 mmol/L	2.12–2.65 mmol/L
Phosphate	3.6 mmol/L	0.8–1.45 mmol/L
Creatine kinase	68,000 IU/L	25–195 IU/L
Arterial blood gases on air		
pH	7.27	7.38–7.44
pco_2	7.5 kPa	4.7–6.0 kPa
po_2	9.2 kPa	12.0–14.5 kPa

Urinalysis: + protein; +++ blood
Urine microscopy: brown urine; no red cells; many granular casts
Electrocardiogram (ECG): flattened P-wave; peaked T-waves
Chest X-ray: extensive left-lower-zone consolidation

Questions
- What is the cause of this patient's acute renal failure?
- What further immediate and longer treatment does this woman need?

ANSWER 44

This patient has acute renal failure as a result of rhabdomyolysis. Severe muscle damage causes a massively elevated serum creatine kinase (CK) level and a rise in serum potassium and phosphate levels. In this case, she has lain unconscious on her left arm for many hours due to an overdose of alcohol and intravenous heroin. As a result, she has developed severe ischaemic muscle damage, causing release of myoglobin, which is toxic to the kidneys. Other causes of rhabdomyolysis include crush injuries, severe hypokalaemia, excessive exercise, myopathies, drugs (e.g. ciclosporin and statins) and certain viral infections. The urine is dark because of the presence of myoglobin, which causes a false-positive dipstick test for blood. Myoglobin has a half-life of 2-3 hours much shorter than CK, and so myoglobinuria has often disappeared whilst the CK is still raised.

Acute renal failure due to rhabdomyolysis causes profound hypocalcaemia in the oliguric phase due to calcium sequestration in muscle and reduced 1,25-dihydroxycalciferol levels, often with rebound hypercalcaemia in the recovery phase. This woman's consciousness level is still depressed as a result of opiate and alcohol toxicity, and she has clinical and radiological evidence of aspiration pneumonia. She has mixed metabolic and respiratory acidosis (low pH, bicarbonate) due to acute renal failure and respiratory depression (pCO$_2$ elevated). Her arterial oxygenation is reduced due to hypoventilation and pneumonia. She also has compartment syndrome in her arm due to massive swelling of her damaged muscles.

This patient has life-threatening hyperkalaemia with electrocardiogram (ECG) changes. The ECG changes of hyperkalaemia progress from the earliest signs of peaking of the T-wave, P-wave flattening, prolongation of the PR interval through to widening of the QRS complex, a sine-wave pattern and ventricular fibrillation. Emergency treatment involves intravenous calcium gluconate, which stabilizes cardiac conduction, and intravenous insulin/glucose, intravenous sodium bicarbonate and nebulized salbutamol, all of which temporarily lower the plasma potassium by increasing the cellular uptake of potassium. However, these steps should be regarded as holding measures while urgent dialysis is being organized.

The chest X-ray and clinical findings indicate consolidation of the left lower lobe. This patient should initially be managed on an intensive care unit. She will require antibiotics for her pneumonia and will require a naloxone infusion or mechanical ventilation for her respiratory failure. The patient should have vigorous rehydration with monitoring of her central venous pressure. If a good urinary flow can be maintained, urinary pH should be kept greater than 7.0 by bicarbonate infusion, which prevents the renal toxicity of myoglobin. This patient also needs to be considered urgently for surgical fasciotomy to relieve the compartment syndrome in her arm.

In the longer term, the patient needs counselling and with her boyfriend should be offered access to drug rehabilitation services. They should also be offered testing for blood-borne viruses (hepatitis B and C and HIV).

 KEY POINTS

- A very high creatine kinase level is diagnostic of rhabdomyolysis. The red/brown urine of myoglobinuria may be absent at presentation because of the speed of clearance of myoglobin.
- As statins are now so widely used, they have become a common cause of rhabdomyolysis, especially when used in high dose and in combination with ciclosporin.
- Aggressive fluid replacement and forced alkaline diuresis can prevent renal damage in rhabdomyolysis if started early enough.

CASE 45: PAINS IN THE ARM

History

A 45-year-old woman makes an appointment to see her general practitioner because of tired-ness. She has found over the past 5 weeks that she has been waking up at night with pain in the right forearm. The pain is relieved a little by taking paracetamol or ibuprofen before going to bed but still disturbs her sleep. She has a history of mild rheumatoid arthritis which has involved her metacarpophalangeal joints, wrists and ankles. This has been controlled since she started taking methotrexate weekly 6 months ago. Over the last week or so she thinks the problem in her right arm is interfering with her work on the computer keyboard.

She works as a secretary and the arthritis had interfered with her work but she has been able to return to work full time since starting the methotrexate.

She has not other relevant medical history. Her mother is on treatment for hypothyroidism and two of her sisters have type 2 diabetes She does not smoke and drinks around 4 units of alcohol a week.

Examination

She weighs 90 kg and her height is 1.68 m. Blood pressure is 132/82 mmHg, pulse 68/min. There is no tenderness or skin abnormality at the site of the pain. She has mild ulnar devia-tion but no tenderness or soft tissue swelling at the metacarpophalangeal joints. There is a little tenderness on resisted movement in both wrists. There is full pain-free movement at her elbow and shoulder joints. On neurological examination there is diminished pinprick and 2 point discrimination in the index and ring fingers of the right hand. Strength in the hand muscles is limited a little by discomfort in the wrist but abduction of the right thumb seems weaker than other movements.

INVESTIGATIONS

		Normal
Haemoglobin	12.5 g/dL	11.7–15.7 g/dL
Mean corpuscular volume (MCV)	102 fL	80–99 fL
White cell count	8.2×10^9/L	$3.5–11.0 \times 10^9$/L
Platelets	350×10^9/L	$150–440 \times 10^9$/L
Sodium	139 mmol/L	135–145 mmol/L
Potassium	4.5 mmol/L	3.5–5.0 mmol/L
Urea	4.4 mmol/L	2.5–6.7 mmol/L
Creatinine	81 µmol/L	70–120 µmol/L
Glucose	4.8 mmol/L	4.0–6.0 mmol/L

Questions

- What is the diagnosis?
- What investigations and treatment would be appropriate?

ANSWER 45

The story of pain in the forearm at night is characteristic of carpal tunnel syndrome caused by compression of the median nerve in the carpal tunnel at the wrist. There are a number of factors in the history that could be related to the reason this woman has developed carpal tunnel syndrome. Rheumatoid arthritis is associated with carpal tunnel syndrome. It is also more likely in those who use their hands at work or other activities. Her return to work as a secretary could be relevant. Other activities such as painting or other do-it-yourself projects may provoke problems. There is a family history of hypothyroidism which is another association. She is obese (BMI 31.9 kg/m^2) which may also be involved. The random blood sugar suggests that she does not have type 2 diabetes as her sisters do, but it would still be sensible to suggest that she tries to lose weight. Women suffer carpal tunnel syndrome more than men. The problem may develop during pregnancy possibly related to fluid retention.

Examination confirms some sensory problems in the distribution of the median nerve and weakness of abductor pollicis brevis in the thenar eminence, supplied by the median nerve. A careful examination is needed to differentiate carpal tunnel syndrome from other neurological problems such as T1 lesions and from weakness associated with active arthritis. Other tests which may help to confirm carpal tunnel syndrome are Tinel's tests where slight percussion over the median nerve provokes tingling in the median nerve distribution and Phalen's manoeuvre where forced flexion at the wrist for 30–60 seconds exacerbates symptoms by increasing compression in the carpal tunnel.

The only significant abnormality in the investigations listed is the raised MCV. This might be related to hypothyroidism and she certainly needs to have her thyroid stimulating hormone (TSH) levels measured. She is on methotrexate and a raised MCV is common on long-term methotrexate therapy. It may indicate folic acid deficiency and there is no indication that she takes folic acid. In addition to TSH she should have measurement of folic acid, vitamin B12 and liver function for investigation of the macrocytosis.

The initial management of her carpal tunnel syndrome is to stop provocative movement temporarily and to give her splints to wear at night. This is usually effective in early cases. If the problems persist then nerve conduction studies will confirm the site and extent of the lesion and local steroid injection or surgical decompression can be considered. In milder cases the outlook is generally good although there may be mild residual tingling.

 KEY POINTS

- Carpal tunnel syndrome often presents with pain at night in the forearm.
- Predisposing causes are hypothyroidism, rheumatoid arthritis, diabetes, acromegaly, obesity and fluid retention as well as repetitive wrist flexion activities and trauma.
- Most cases settle without surgical intervention.

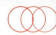

CASE 46: NAUSEA AND VERTIGO

History

A 17-year-old woman is admitted to the emergency department complaining of severe vertigo. This has developed over the past few hours, and previously she was well. She has the sensation of her surroundings spinning around her. She feels nauseated and sleepy. She does not have a headache. She has not had any previous medical illnesses. She is a non-smoker and says that she does not drink alcohol or take recreational drugs, and she is taking no regular medication. She lives with her parents and is due to sit her A-levels in 3 weeks. Her father suffers from epilepsy, and her mother has hypothyroidism.

Examination

She is drowsy, and her speech is slurred. Her pulse rate is 64/min, blood pressure is 90/70 mmHg, and respiratory rate is 12/min. Examination of her cardiovascular, respiratory and abdominal systems is otherwise normal. Her peripheral nervous system examination is normal apart from impaired coordination in both arms and legs and a staggering gait. Fundoscopy is normal. Her pupils are equal and reacting. There is a normal range of eye movements, but she has multidirectional nystagmus. Her hearing is normal, as is the rest of her cranial nerve examination.

Questions
- What is the diagnosis?
- What are the major differential diagnoses of vertigo?
- How would you manage this patient?

ANSWER 46

The acute onset of these symptoms and signs with drowsiness in a 17-year-old girl raises the possibility of a drug overdose. Her father is epileptic and is likely to be taking anticonvulsants. The most likely explanation is that this patient has taken a phenytoin overdose, tablets that her father uses to control his epilepsy. She may have taken an overdose because of concern about her imminent exams. Excessive ingestion of barbiturates, alcohol and phenytoin all cause acute neurotoxicity manifested by vertigo, dysarthria, ataxia and nystagmus. In severe cases coma, respiratory depression and hypotension occur.

Vertigo is an awareness of disordered orientation of the body in space and takes the form of a sensation of rotation of the body or its surroundings.

! Causes of vertigo

Peripheral lesions	Central lesions
Benign positional vertigo	Brainstem ischaemia
Vestibular neuronitis	Posterior fossa tumours
Ménière's disease	Multiple sclerosis
Middle-ear diseases	Alcohol/drugs
Aminoglycoside toxicity	Migraine, epilepsy

The duration of attacks is helpful in distinguishing some of these causes of vertigo. Benign positional vertigo lasts less than 1 min. Attacks of Ménière's disease are recurrent and last up to 24 h. Vestibular neuronitis does not recur but lasts several days, whereas vertigo due to ototoxic drugs is usually permanent. Brainstem ischaemic attacks occur in patients with evidence of diffuse vascular disease, and long tract signs may be present. Multiple sclerosis may initially present with an acute attack of vertigo that lasts for 2–3 weeks. Posterior fossa tumours usually have symptoms and signs of space-occupying lesions. Acoustic neuromas often present with vertigo and deafness. Migrainous attacks are often accompanied by nausea and vomiting. Temporal lobe epilepsy may also produce rotational vertigo, often associated with auditory and visual hallucinations. Central lesions produce nystagmus, which is multi-directional and may be vertical. Peripheral lesions induce a unilateral horizontal nystagmus.

The diagnosis in this case can be made by measuring plasma phenytoin levels and by asking the patient's father to check if his tablets are missing. Gastric lavage should be carried out if it is within 12 h of ingestion of the tablets. Oral activated charcoal may be useful. National poison information services are available to advise on treatment. Before discharge she should be assessed and have counselling and treatment by psychiatrists specializing in adolescents.

 KEY POINTS

- Vertigo can be caused by a variety of neurological disorders.
- A careful history and examination may reveal the cause of vertigo.
- Overdose should be considered in any patient presenting with decreased consciousness level and respiratory depression.

CASE 47: CHEST PAIN

History
A 64-year-old woman has a 10-year history of retrosternal pain. The pain is often present in bed at night and may be precipitated by bending down. Occasionally, the pain comes on after eating, and on some occasions it appears to have been precipitated by exercise. The pain has been described as having a burning and a tight quality to it. The pain is not otherwise exacerbated by respiratory movements or position.

Her husband has angina, and on one occasion she took one of his glyceryl trinitrate tablets. She thinks that this probably helped her pain since it seemed to stop a little faster than usual. She has also bought some indigestion tablets from a local pharmacy and thinks that these probably helped also.

Examination
She is 1.62 m (5 ft 4 in.) tall and weighs 82 kg, giving her a body mass index of 31.3 kg/m² (recommended range 20–25 kg/m²) No abnormalities are found in the cardiovascular, respiratory or gastrointestinal systems.

🔍 INVESTIGATIONS

- Her chest X-ray is normal, and the electrocardiogram is shown in Figure 47.1.
- She had an exercise electrocardiogram (ECG) performed, and she was able to perform 8 min of exercise. Her heart rate went up to 130/min with no change in the ST segments on the ECG and normal heart and blood pressure responses.
- The haemoglobin, renal and liver functions are normal.

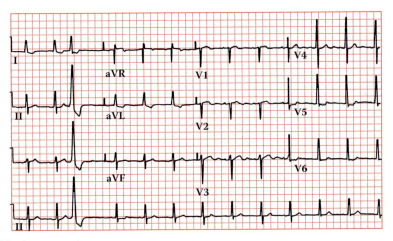

Figure 47.1 Electrocardiogram.

Questions
- What is the likely diagnosis?
- What would be appropriate management?

ANSWER 47

A number of features in the history make oesophageal reflux a likely diagnosis. The character and position of the pain and the relation to lying flat and to bending mean reflux is more likely. She is overweight, increasing the likelihood of reflux. The improvement with glyceryl trinitrate and with proprietary antacids is inconclusive. The ECG shows one ventricular ectopic and some T-wave changes in leads I, aVl, V5 and V6, which would be compatible with myocardial ischaemia but are not specific. The exercise ECG was negative, which reduces the likelihood of ischaemic heart disease, although it certainly does not rule it out. Other causes of chest pain are less likely with the length of history.

In view of the long history and the features suggesting oesophageal reflux, it would be reasonable to initiate a trial of therapy for oesophageal reflux with regular antacid therapy, H_2-receptor blockers or a proton pump inhibitor (omeprazole or lansoprazole). If the pain responds to this form of therapy, then additional actions such as weight loss (she is well above ideal body weight) and raising the head of the bed at night should be added. If doubt remains, a barium swallow should show the tendency to reflux, and a gastroscopy would show evidence of oesophagitis. There is a broad association between the presence of oesophageal reflux, evidence of oesophagitis at endoscopy and biopsy, and the symptoms of heartburn. However, each can occur independently of the others.

Recording of pH in the oesophagus over 24 h can provide additional useful information. It is achieved by passing a small pH-sensitive electrode into the oesophagus through the nose. This provides an objective measure of the amount of acid reaching the oesophagus and the times when this occurs.

This woman had an endoscopy that showed oesophagitis, and treatment with omeprazole and an alginate relieved her symptoms. Attempts at weight loss were not successful.

 KEY POINTS

- In non-specific chest pain with a normal ECG, the oesophagus is a common source of the pain.
- A 24-h pH recording in the oesophagus provides further information on acid reflux.

CASE 48: HEADACHES

History

A 44-year-old woman presents to her general practitioner (GP) complaining of headaches. These headaches have been present in previous years but have now become more intense. She describes the headaches as severe and present on both sides of her head. They tend to worsen during the course of the day. There is no associated visual disturbance or vomiting. She also complains of loss of appetite and difficulty sleeping, with early morning waking. She has had eczema and irritable bowel syndrome diagnosed in the past, but these are not giving her problems at the moment. She is divorced with two children, aged 10 and 12 years, whom she looks after. She has a part-time job as an office cleaner. Her mother has recently died of a brain tumour. She smokes about 20 cigarettes per day and drinks 15 units of alcohol per week. She takes regular paracetamol or ibuprofen for her headaches.

Examination

She looks withdrawn. Her pulse is 74/min and regular; blood pressure is 118/76 mmHg. Examination of the cardiovascular, respiratory and gastrointestinal systems, breasts and reticuloendothelial system is normal. There are no abnormal neurological signs, and funduscopy is normal.

Questions
- What is the diagnosis?
- What are the major differential diagnoses?
- How would you manage this patient?

ANSWER 48

This patient has a chronic tension headache. This is the commonest form of headache. It occurs mainly in patients under the age of 50 years. The headache is usually bilateral, often with diffuse radiation over the vertex of the skull, although it may be more localized. The pain is often characterized as a sense of pressure on the head. Visual symptoms and vomiting do not occur. The pain is often at its worst in the evening. Patients may show symptoms of depression (this woman has biological symptoms of loss of appetite and disturbed sleep pattern). Sufferers may reveal sources of stress such as bereavement or difficulty with work. There may be an element of suggestion as in this case, with concern that she may have inherited a brain tumour from her mother. She is looking after two children alone and working part-time. A normal neurological examination is important for reassurance.

! **Major differential diagnoses of chronic headaches**

- *Classic migraine*: characterized by visual symptoms followed within 30 min by the onset of severe hemicranial throbbing, headache, photophobia, nausea and vomiting lasting for several hours. The onset is usually in early adult life, and a positive family history may be present.
- *Cluster headaches*: mainly affect men. The pain is unilateral, usually orbital and severe in nature. It characteristically occurs 1–2 h after sleeping, lasts 1–2 h, and recurs nightly for 6–8 weeks.
- *Headache caused by a space-occupying lesion* (such as tumour or abscess): Often the headache is initially mild, but over a few weeks becomes severe and is exacerbated by coughing or sneezing. The headache is usually worse in the morning and is associated with vomiting. There will often be other signs, including personality change and focal neurological signs.
- *Miscellaneous causes*: sinusitis, dental disorders, cervical spondylosis, glaucoma, post-traumatic headache.

It is important to come to a clear diagnosis and to address the patient's beliefs and concerns about the symptoms. In some circumstances it may be necessary to perform a computed tomography (CT) head scan for reassurance. The question of depression needs to be explored further and may need treating with antidepressants.

 KEY POINTS

- Tension headaches occur mainly in those aged under 50, and patients often show features of depression.
- Tension headache should be diagnosed after other causes have been excluded.

CASE 49: HEADACHE AND CONFUSION

History

A 55-year-old man is admitted to hospital with headache and confusion. He has a cough and a temperature of 38.2°C. He does not complain of any other symptoms. Two months earlier he had been admitted with a productive cough, and acid-fast bacilli had been found in the sputum on direct smear. He had lost weight and complained of occasional night sweats. He had a history of a head injury 10 years previously. He smoked 15 cigarettes a day and drank 40–60 units of alcohol each week. He was found a place in a local hostel for the homeless and sent out after 1 week in hospital on antituberculous treatment with rifampicin, isoniazid, ethambutol and pyrazinamide together with pyridoxine. His chest X-ray at the time was reported as showing probable infiltration in the right upper lobe.

Examination

He looked thin and unwell, and he was slightly drowsy. His mini-mental test score was 8/10. There were some crackles in the upper zones of the chest posteriorly. His respiratory rate was 22/min. There were no neurological signs.

 INVESTIGATIONS

His chest X-ray is shown in Figure 49.1.

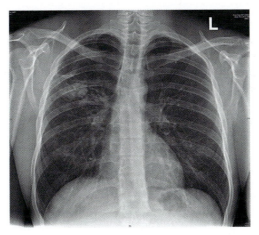

Figure 49.1 Chest X-ray.

Question
- What might be the cause of his second admission?

ANSWER 49

The chest X-ray shows extensive changes in the right upper zone that seem as if they are likely to be more extensive than those described at the first admission 2 months earlier. It is likely that this is a worsening of his pulmonary tuberculosis. This might have occurred because he had a resistant organism or, more likely, because he had not taken his treatment as prescribed. Risk factors for development of tuberculosis are poor nutrition, high alcohol intake and immunosuppression (HIV, immunosuppressive therapy). Higher rates occur in those from the Indian subcontinent and parts of Africa.

The headache and confusion raise the possibility of tuberculous meningitis. Other possibilities would be liver damage from the antituberculous drugs and the alcohol, although clinical jaundice would be expected, or hyponatraemia or hypercalcaemia. If these are not present a lumbar puncture would be indicated if there is no sign to suggest raised intracranial pressure. It would be advisable to do a computed tomography (CT) scan of the brain first since a fall related to his high alcohol consumption might have led to a subdural haemorrhage to give him his headache and confusion.

It is now 2 months since the initial finding of acid-fast bacilli in the sputum, and the cultures and sensitivities of the organism should be available. These should be checked to be sure that the organism was *Mycobacterium tuberculosis,* and that it was sensitive to the four antituberculous drugs he was given. As a check on compliance, blood levels of antituberculous drugs can be measured. The urine will be coloured orangey-red by metabolites of rifampicin taken in the previous 8 h or so.

Comparison with his old chest X-rays showed extension of the right upper-lobe shadowing. It is difficult to be sure about activity from a chest X-ray, but extension of shadowing is obviously suspicious. 'Softer', fluffier shadowing is more likely to be associated with active disease. A direct smear of the sputum showed that acid-fast bacilli were still present on direct smear. He confirmed that he was not taking his medication regularly. His headache and confusion resolved as he stopped his high alcohol intake. Subsequently the antituberculous therapy should be given as directly observed therapy (DOT) in a thrice-weekly regime supervised at each administration by a district nurse or health visitor.

 KEY POINTS

- Poor adherence to treatment regimes is the commonest cause of failure of antituberculous and other treatment.
- Directly observed therapy should be used when there is any doubt about likely adherence to treatment.
- Initial polymerase chain reaction testing on sputum can predict the likelihood of resistant organisms.

CASE 50: CHEST PAIN AND SHORTNESS OF BREATH

History

A 29-year-old woman complained of a sudden onset of right-sided chest pain with shortness of breath. It woke her from sleep at 3:00 am. The pain was made worse by a deep breath and by coughing. The breathlessness persisted over the 4h from its onset to her arrival in the emergency department. She has a slight non-productive cough. There is no relevant previous medical history except asthma controlled by salbutamol and beclometasone. There is no family history of note. She works as a driving instructor and had returned from a 3-week holiday in Australia 3 weeks previously. She had no illnesses while she was away. She has taken an oral contraceptive for the last 4 years.

Examination

She has a temperature of 37.4°C, her respiratory rate is 24/min, the jugular venous pressure is raised 3 cm, the blood pressure is 110/64 mmHg, and the pulse rate is 128/min. Peak flow rate is 410 L/min. In the respiratory system, expansion is reduced because of pain. Percussion and tactile vocal fremitus are normal and equal. A pleural rub can be heard over the right lower zone posteriorly. There are no other added sounds. Otherwise the examination is normal.

🔍 **INVESTIGATIONS**

- An electrocardiogram (ECG) is shown in Figure 50.1.
- Figure 50.2 shows her chest X-ray.

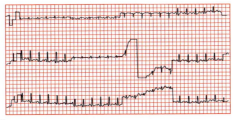

Figure 50.1 Electrocardiogram.

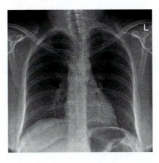

Figure 50.2 Chest X-ray.

Questions

- What is the likely diagnosis?
- How can it be confirmed?

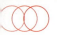

ANSWER 50

This woman has had a sudden onset of pleuritic pain, breathlessness and cough. The physical signs of tachypnoea, tachycardia, raised jugular venous pressure and pleural rub would fit with a diagnosis of a pulmonary embolus. The peak flow of 410 L/min indicates that asthma does not explain her breathlessness.

The differential diagnosis would include pneumonia, pneumothorax and pulmonary embolism. The clinical signs do not suggest pneumothorax or pneumonia. Possible pre-disposing factors for pulmonary embolism are the history of a long aeroplane journey 3 weeks earlier, oral contraception and her work involving sitting for prolonged periods. Other predisposing factors, such as intravenous drug abuse, should be considered. The ECG shows sinus tachycardia. The often-quoted pattern of S-wave in lead I, Q-wave and T inversion in lead III (S1Q3T3) is not common except with massive pulmonary embolus. Other signs, such as transient right ventricular hypertrophy features, P pulmonale and T-wave changes, may also occur. The chest X-ray is normal, ruling out pneumothorax and lobar pneumonia.

A ventilation–perfusion lung scan could be done looking for a typical mismatch with an area that is ventilated but not perfused. This result would have a high probability for a diagnosis of pulmonary embolism. A pulmonary arteriogram has been the 'gold standard' for the diagnosis of embolism but is a more invasive test. In cases with a normal chest X-ray and no history of chronic lung disease, equivocal results are less common, and it is not usually necessary to go further than the lung scan. In the presence of chronic lung disease such as chronic obstructive pulmonary disease (COPD) or significant asthma, the ventilation–perfusion lung scan is more likely to be equivocal, and further tests are more often used. In this case a computed tomography (CT) pulmonary angiogram was carried out (Figure 50.3). This showed a filling defect typical of an embolus in the right lower lobe pulmonary artery.

A search for a source of emboli with a Doppler of the leg veins may help in some cases, and the finding of negative D-dimers in the blood makes intravascular thrombosis and embolism unlikely.

Immediate management should involve heparin, usually as subcutaneous low-molecular-weight heparin. The anticoagulation can then transfer to warfarin, continued in a case like this for 6 months. Alternative modes of contraception should be discussed and advice given on alternating walking or other leg movements with her seated periods at work. Thrombolysis should be considered when there is haemodynamic compromise by a large embolus.

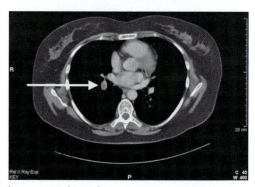

Figure 50.3 Computed tomography pulmonary angiogram.

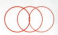

 KEY POINTS

- In the presence of a normal chest X-ray and no chronic lung disease, the ventilation–perfusion lung scan has good sensitivity and specificity.
- The chest X-ray and ECG are often unhelpful in the diagnosis of pulmonary embolism.
- CT pulmonary arteriogram is used when ventilation–perfusion scanning is likely to be unhelpful.

CASE 51: CHEST PAIN

History

A 62-year-old man is admitted to hospital with chest pain. The pain is in the centre of the chest and has lasted for 3 h by the time of his arrival in the emergency department. The chest pain radiated to the jaw and left shoulder. He felt sick at the same time. He has a history of chest pain on exercise, which has been present for 6 months. He has smoked 10 cigarettes daily for 40 years and does not drink alcohol. He has been treated with aspirin and with beta-blockers regularly for the last 2 years and has been given a glyceryl trinitrate spray to use as needed. This turns out to be two or three times a week. His father died of a myocardial infarction at age 66 years, and his 65-year-old brother had a coronary artery bypass graft 4 years ago.

He has no other previous medical history. He works as a security guard.

Examination

He is sweaty and in pain but has no abnormalities in the cardiovascular or respiratory systems. His blood pressure is 138/82 mmHg, and his pulse rate is 110/min and regular.

 INVESTIGATIONS

His electrocardiogram (ECG) is shown in Figure 51.1.

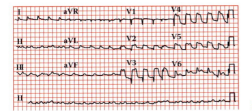

Figure 51.1 Electrocardiogram.

He was given analgesia and underwent emergency primary angioplasty and stenting to a severe left anterior coronary artery lesion, and clopidrogel was added to his treatment. His pain settled and after two days he began to mobilize. On the fourth day after admission, he became more unwell.

On examination, now his jugular venous pressure is raised to 6 cm above the manubriosternal angle. His blood pressure is 102/64 mmHg; pulse rate is 106/min and regular. His temperature is 37.8°C. On auscultation of the heart, there is a loud systolic murmur heard all over the praecordium. In the respiratory system, there are late inspiratory crackles at the lung bases, and these are heard up to the midzones. There are no new abnormalities to find elsewhere on examination. His chest X-ray is shown in Figure 51.2.

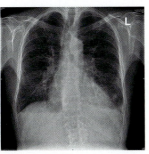

Figure 51.2 Chest X-ray.

Questions

- What is the likely diagnosis?
- How might this be confirmed?

ANSWER 51

This 62-year-old man had an anteroseptal myocardial infarction, indicated by Q-waves in V2 and V3 and raised ST segments in V2, V3, V4 and V5. He became unwell suddenly 4 days later having had no initial problems. The late inspiratory crackles are typical of pulmonary oedema, and the chest X-ray confirms this, showing hilar flare with some alveolar filling, Kerley B lines at the lung bases and blunting of the costophrenic angles with small pleural effusions.

The problems likely to occur at this time and produce shortness of breath are a further myocardial infarction, arrhythmias, rupture of the chordae tendinae of the mitral valve, perforation of the intraventricular septum or even the free wall of the ventricle, and pulmonary emboli. The first four of these could produce pulmonary oedema and a raised jugular venous pressure, as in this man. Pulmonary embolism would be compatible with a raised jugular venous pressure but not the findings of pulmonary oedema on examination and X-ray.

Acute mitral regurgitation from chordal rupture and ischaemic perforation of the interventricular septum both produce a loud pansystolic murmur. The site of maximum intensity of the murmur may differ, being apical with chordal rupture and at the lower left sternal edge with ventricular septal defect, but this differentiation may not be possible with a loud murmur. The differentiation can be made by echocardiography.

The management of acute ventricular septal defect or chordal rupture would be similar and should involve consultation with the cardiac surgeons. When these lesions produce haemodynamic problems, as in this case, surgical repair is needed, either acutely if the problem is very severe or after stabilization with antifailure treatment or even counterpulsation with an aortic balloon pump. Milder degrees of failure with a pansystolic murmur may occur when there is ischaemia of the papillary muscles of the mitral valve. This is managed with antifailure treatment, not surgical intervention, and can be differentiated by echocardiography.

 KEY POINTS

- The cause of breathlessness after myocardial infarction needs careful evaluation.
- The signs of ischaemic ventricular septal defect and mitral regurgitation due to chordal rupture after myocardial infarction may be very difficult to differentiate.
- Patients with angina or myocardial infarction can also present with the radiating pain but no central chest pain or with only the cardiac effects and no pain at all.

CASE 52: GENERAL WEAKNESS

History
An 82-year-old man is sent to the emergency department by his general practitioner (GP). The man is complaining of weakness and general malaise. He has complained of general pains in the muscles, and he also has some pains in the joints, particularly the elbows, wrists and knees. Three weeks earlier, he fell and hit his leg and has some local pain related to this.

He is a non-smoker who does not drink any alcohol and has not been on any medication. Twelve years ago he had a myocardial infarction and was put on a beta-blocker, but he has not had a prescription for this in the last 6 years. Twenty years ago he had a cholecystectomy. He used to work as a labourer until his retirement at the age of 63 years.

He lives alone in a second-floor flat. His wife died 5 years ago. He has one son who lives in Ireland and whom he has not seen for 3 years.

Examination
He is tender over the muscles around his limb girdles, and there is a little tenderness over the elbows, wrists and knees. The mouth looks normal except that his tongue appears rather smooth. He has no teeth and has lost his dentures. There are no other abnormalities to find in the cardiovascular, respiratory or alimentary systems. In the legs, he has a superficial laceration on the front of the right shin. This is oozing blood and has not healed. There is a petechial rash around the ankles. There are some larger areas of bruising on the arms and the legs, which he says have not been associated with any trauma.

INVESTIGATIONS

		Normal
Haemoglobin	10.1 g/dL	13.7–17.7 g/dL
Mean corpuscular volume (MCV)	74 fL	80–99 fL
White cell count	7.9×10^9/L	$3.9–10.6 \times 10^9$/L
Neutrophils	6.3×10^9/L	$1.8–7.7 \times 10^9$/L
Lymphocytes	1.2×10^9/L	$1.0–4.8 \times 10^9$/L
Platelets	334×10^9/L	$150–440 \times 10^9$/L

Questions
- What essential area of the history is not covered?
- What is the likely diagnosis?

ANSWER 52

A dietary history is an essential part of any history and is particularly important here; a number of features point towards a possible nutritional problem. He has been a widower for 5 years with no family support. He lives alone on a second-floor flat, which may make it difficult for him to get out. He has lost his dentures, which is likely to make it difficult for him to eat. The easiest way may be to ask him to tell you what he eats in a typical day and his food intake in the last 48 hours.

He has a petechial rash, which could be related to coagulation problems, but the platelet count is normal. It would be important to examine the rash carefully to see if it is distributed around the hair follicles. A number of the features suggest a possible diagnosis of scurvy from vitamin C deficiency. Body stores of vitamin C are sufficient to last 2–3 months. The rash, muscle and joint pains and tenderness, poor wound healing and microcytic anaemia are all features of scurvy. The classic feature of bleeding from the gums would not be present in an edentulous patient.

Plasma measurements of vitamin C are difficult because of the wide range in normal subjects. In this patient, replacement with ascorbic acid orally cleared up the symptoms within 2 weeks. It would be important to look for other nutritional deficiencies in this situation and to arrange support to ensure that the situation did not recur after his discharge from hospital.

 KEY POINTS

- A nutritional history should be part of any clinical assessment, particularly in the elderly.
- Vitamin deficiencies can occur in patients on a poor diet in the absence of any problem with malabsorption.

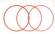

CASE 53: LOSS OF CONSCIOUSNESS

History

An unkempt man of uncertain age, estimated to be 55–65 years, is brought to hospital by ambulance, having been found unconscious on the pavement outside a pub on New Year's Eve. There is no other available history. A used packet of paracetamol and dihydrocodeine is found in one of his pockets, but no illicit drugs and no means of identification are found.

On examination he looks pale and smells of alcohol and urine. There are no signs of head injury and no localizing neurological signs.

Examination

Tendon reflexes are present and equal except the ankle reflexes, which are absent. Plantar responses are downgoing. The pupils are equal and reactive, and the fundi look normal. The observation chart is completed by the nurse in the emergency department.

🔍 INVESTIGATIONS

- Pulse: 82/min
- Blood pressure: 92/56 mmHg
- Temperature: 35.1°C
- Respiratory rate: 12/min
- Oxygen saturation: 95 per cent breathing air
- Glasgow Coma Scale: 10/15
- Urine on catheterization: 450 mL volume; + sugar; + blood; no protein

The electrocardiogram (ECG) is shown in Figure 53.1..

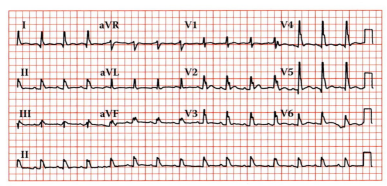

Figure 53.1 Electrocardiogram.

Questions

- What is the likely cause of the problem?
- What investigations and treatment are indicated?

ANSWER 53

This man has been unconscious in the open air for an unknown period. Little history is available, but the tablets in his pocket might suggest that he has a problem with a painful condition. There are a number of possible causes for his unconsciousness, including a cerebrovascular problem; deliberate or accidental drug overdose, including alcohol poisoning; metabolic or endocrine disturbance; or hypothermia.

If this were an overdose (e.g. of dihydrocodeine), the pupils might well be small. The slow respiratory rate could be compatible with an opiate excess suppressing ventilation. The oxygen saturation results show that he is oxygenating himself satisfactorily, although it would be sensible to perform blood gases to measure the arterial partial pressure of CO_2 ($PaCO_2$). It would be appropriate to measure the paracetamol level in the blood, and it would be worth giving the opiate antagonist naloxone if there remained a likelihood of overdose. The blood alcohol level should be measured to exclude alcohol poisoning.

Most cerebrovascular problems would be expected to produce some localizing neurological signs on careful examination, even in an unconscious patient. There are no such signs here. The absent ankle jerks might be related to his age.

He could have hyperosmolar non-ketotic coma detected by a high glucose and evidence of haemoconcentration. The blood glucose should be measured together with electrolytes and haematology, but the single plus sign of glucose in the urine makes it unlikely that he has hyperglycaemic coma. Liver function and renal function should be measured.

He has a slow respiratory rate, low blood pressure and an ECG that shows a wide QRS complex. The wide complexes on the ECG show an extra deflection at the end of the QRS complex, the J point. This J-wave is characteristic of hypothermia and disappears after rewarming, as shown by the subsequent ECG (Figure 53.2). The pulse rate would often be slower than the 82/min in this man, and the ECG may show evidence of a tremor from shivering. The temperature of 35.1°C does not appear excessively low, but this may not be reliable if it is not a true core temperature or has been measured with a normal mercury thermometer (mercury thermometers are not reliable at low temperatures). Indeed, in this case, repeat of the rectal temperature measurement with a low-reading thermometer showed a temperature of 30.6°C. No paracetamol was detected in the blood, and his alcohol level was low at 11 mg/100 mL.

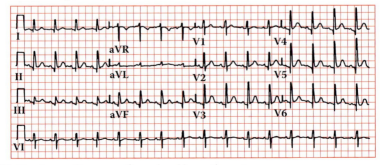

Figure 53.2 Electrocardiogram of resolved hypothermia.

The management of hypothermia is gradual passive rewarming with replacement of fluids by warmed colloids as rewarming takes place. The increase of temperature should be 0.5–1°C per hour. If this is not achieved by covering the patient with blankets, then warmed inspired oxygen, warm intravenous fluids, bladder or peritoneal lavage might be considered. Drugs and physical disturbance should be limited since the myocardium is often irritable and susceptible to arrhythmias.

KEY POINTS

- Hypothyroidism should be considered as a possible contributor to hypothermia.
- Even when alcohol is a cause of unconsciousness, other causes must be excluded.
- The diagnosis of hypothermia requires a thermometer capable of reading low temperatures.
- J-waves on the ECG are specific signs of hypothermia.
- Hypothermia in the elderly is treated by gradual passive rewarming.

CASE 54: TIREDNESS

History

A 22-year-old woman complains of tiredness for 6 months. Her only other symptom is a gradual increase in frequency of bowel movements from once a day in her teens to two to three times daily. She has no abdominal pain and has no change in appetite. She says that the bowel movements can be difficult to flush away on occasions, but this is not a consistent problem. She is a non-smoker and drinks rarely. She has been a vegetarian for 5 years but eats dairy foods and fish regularly. She thinks that her grandmother, who lived in Ireland, had some bowel problems, but she died 3 years ago, at aged 68. She is an infant-school teacher and spends a lot of her spare time in keep-fit classes and routines at a local gym. She enjoys her work and socializes regularly with a wide circle of friends.

Examination

She is 1.62 m (5 ft 4 in.) tall and weighs 49 kg. She looks a little pale and thin. Examination of her abdomen showed no abnormalities, and there are no other significant abnormalities to find in any other system.

INVESTIGATIONS

		Normal
Haemoglobin	9.8 g/dL	11.7–15.7 g/dL
Mean corpuscular volume (MCV)	98 fL	80–99 fL
White cell count	6.5×10^9/L	$3.5–11.0 \times 10^9$/L
Platelets	247×10^9/L	$150–440 \times 10^9$/L
Red cell folate	44 mg/L	>160 mg/L
Vitamin B_{12}	280 ng/L	176–925 ng/L
Thyroid-stimulating hormone	3.5 mU/L	0.3–6.0 mU/L
Free thyroxine	12.9 pmol/L	9.0–22.0 pmol/L

The blood film is reported as a dimorphic film with remnants of nuclear material (Howell–Jolly bodies) in some of the red blood cells.

Questions

- How do you interpret these findings?
- What is the likely diagnosis, and how might this be confirmed?

ANSWER 54

The most likely diagnosis is malabsorption from coeliac disease. The report of a dimorphic blood film means that there are both small and large cells. This suggests that the anaemia is caused by a combination of the folate deficiency indicated by the red cell folate and by iron deficiency. The Howell–Jolly bodies are dark blue regular inclusions in the red cells that are typically found in the blood of patients after splenectomy or are associated with the splenic atrophy characteristic of coeliac disease. In coeliac disease, there is a sensitivity to dietary gluten, a water-insoluble protein found in many cereals. The proximal small bowel is the main site involved with loss of villi and an inflammatory infiltrate causing reduced absorption.

The MCV is at the upper limit of normal.

> **!** **Causes of macrocytosis in the blood film**
> - Folate deficiency
> - Vitamin B_{12} deficiency
> - Excessive alcohol consumption
> - Hypothyroidism
> - Certain drugs (e.g. azathioprine, methotrexate)
> - Primary acquired sideroblastic anaemia and myelodysplastic syndromes

Coeliac disease is made more likely by a possible positive family history and the origin from Ireland, where coeliac disease is four times as common as in the rest of the United Kingdom. Other diagnoses that might be considered are anorexia nervosa (her age and sex, commitment to exercise); she does not appear depressed (a common cause of weight loss and bowel disturbance), and the laboratory findings clearly indicate physical disease.

Diagnosis of coeliac disease can be confirmed by endoscopy, at which a biopsy can be taken from the distal duodenum. Typically this will show complete villus atrophy. IgA anti-tissue transglutaminase and IgA endomysial antibodies are usually positive when the patient is still in a gluten containing diet and are a useful screening test. Treatment is a gluten-free diet with a repeat of the biopsy some months later to show improvement in the height of the villi in the small bowel. In some cases, temporary treatment with steroids may be needed to help recovery. A common cause of failure to recover the villus architecture is poor compliance to the difficult dietary constraints. Symptoms may persist if patients have lactose intolerance or irritable bowel syndrome.

> **KEY POINTS**
> - Howell–Jolly bodies are characteristic of hyposplenism.
> - Coeliac disease can present at any age with non-specific symptoms; absence of abdominal pain or steatorrhoea are not unusual.
> - Typical features of fat malabsorption may not be evident if the patient eats a diet with little or no fat intake.

CASE 55: RECURRENT CHEST INFECTIONS

History

A 45-year-old woman is admitted to hospital with pneumonia. She has had three episodes of cough, fever and purulent sputum over the last 6 months. One of these was associated with right-sided pleuritic chest pain. These have been treated at home by her general practitioner (GP). In addition she has a 5-year history of difficulty with swallowing. Initially this was mild, but it has become progressively worse. She says that food seems to stick in the low retrosternal area. This applies to all types of solid food. She has lost 5 kg in weight over the last 2 months. Sometimes the difficulty with swallowing seems to improve during a meal. Recently she has had trouble with regurgitation and vomiting of recognizable food.

Three years ago her GP arranged for an outpatient upper gastrointestinal endoscopy, which was normal. She was reassured, but the problem has increased in severity. There is no other relevant medical history or family history. She lived in the north-western coast of the United States for 4 years until 10 years ago. She works as a shop assistant. She has never smoked and drinks less than 5 units of alcohol each week. There has been no disturbance of micturition. She has always tended to be constipated, and this has been a little worse recently.

Examination

She looks thin. In the respiratory system there are some crackles at the right base. There are no abnormalities in the cardiovascular system, abdomen or other systems.

 INVESTIGATIONS

Her chest X-ray is shown in Figure 55.1.

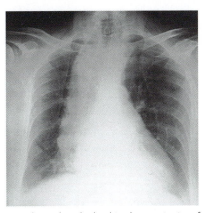

Figure 55.1 Chest X-ray. (Reproduced with the kind permission from Curtis and Whitehouse, *Radiology for the MRCP*, Arnold, London, 1998.)

Questions

- What is the likely diagnosis?
- How would you establish this?

ANSWER 55

The likely diagnosis is achalasia of the cardia, a primary neurological disturbance of the nerve plexuses at the lower end of the oesophagus. The X-ray shows a dilated, fluid-filled oesophagus with no visible gastric air bubble. Endoscopy may be normal in the early stages, as in this case. The oesophagus has now dilated, and there has been spillover of stagnant food into the lungs, giving her the episodes of repeated respiratory infections. Such aspiration is most likely to affect the right lower lobe because of the more vertical right main bronchus, although the result of aspiration at night may depend on the position of the patient. The dysphagia is often variable early on. It tends to be present for all foods, indicating a motility problem, and there may initially be some relief from the mechanical load as the oesophagus fills. Dysphagia for bulky, solid foods first usually indicates an obstructive lesion.

The diagnosis can be made at this stage by a barium swallow showing the dilated oesophagus. Earlier, it may require careful cine-radiology with a bolus of food impregnated with barium or oesophageal motility studies using a catheter fitted with a number of pressure sensors to detect the abnormal motility of the oesophageal muscle.

A similar condition can be produced by the protozoan parasite *Trypanosoma cruzi* (Chagas' disease), but this is limited to South and Central America and would not be relevant to her stay in the north-western United States.

Other common causes of dysphagia are benign oesophageal structures from acid reflux, malignant structures, external compression or an oesophageal pouch. Achalasia may be managed by muscle relaxants when mild, but often requires treatment to disrupt the lower oesophageal muscle by endoscopic dilation or surgery.

 KEY POINTS

- The subjective site of blockage in dysphagia may not reflect accurately the level of the obstruction.
- Persistent dysphagia without explanation needs investigation by barium swallow or endoscopy.

CASE 56: HEADACHE

History

A 74-year-old woman presents as an emergency having suddenly developed a severe head-ache whilst shovelling snow in her drive. She does not recollect being taken to the hospital. The ambulance was called by the neighbours who witnessed the woman having generalised seizures. She now describes the pain as the worst headache that she has ever experienced. It is a generalised headache. She cannot tolerate bright light. She had a similar milder head-ache about 10 days earlier. She has a history of well-controlled hypertension. She smokes 20 cigarettes/day.

Examination

On examination she was drowsy. There was marked neck stiffness and photophobia. Blood pressure was 172/102. There were no focal neurological signs.

Questions

- What is the likely diagnosis?
- What are the major differential diagnoses?
- How would you investigate this patient?

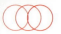

ANSWER 56

Headache is one of the commonest clinical complaints. The sudden onset of a headache within seconds or a few minutes is characteristic of a subarachnoid haemaorrhage (SAH). In contrast a migraine usually takes one to two hours to reach maximal intensity. The absence of a similar headache in the past also suggests a new pathology.

Tension type headaches are the commonest headaches in the general population. The typical presentation is of mild to moderate headache, nonthrobbing, bilateral with no associated symptoms. Cluster headaches are characterised by attacks of severe unilateral orbital or temporal pain, accompanied by autonomic features such as nasal congestion, lacrimation and rhinorrhoea. Migraines are often preceded by characteristic symptoms such as flashing lights and are often unilateral. Nausea and photophobia may occur during an attack. Brain tumours cause headaches by causing raised intracranial pressure. The headache is worse after coughing and is often associated with nausea and vomiting.

Patients with SAH often describe the pain as 'the worst headache in my life'. Fever associated with headache suggests an infective cause such as meningitis. A change in conscious level or personality suggests an underlying pathology. Rupture of an aneurysm leads to release of blood into the cerebrospinal fluid (CSF) under arterial pressure. The bleeding probably only lasts for a few seconds, but rebleeding is common. The onset of headache may be localised to the side of the aneurysm and may be associated with a brief loss of consciousness, seizure, nausea and vomiting and neck stiffness. A significant minority of patients will have a minor haemorrhage causing a sudden and severe headache (the sentinel headache) within the 3 weeks leading up to the main SAH. Physical exertion may be a trigger. Risk factors include smoking, heavy alcohol consumption, uncontrolled hypertension and a family history.

On examination, conscious level may be reduced. There is neck stiffness and there may be preretinal haemorrhages. The key investigation is a noncontrast CT scan. The sensitivity of a head CT for detecting blood in the CSF is highest in the first 6–12 hours, and then declines rapidly over the next few days. Lumbar puncture is essential if there is a high clinical suspicion of a SAH haemorrhage with a normal CT. The usual findings are an elevated opening pressure and an elevated red blood cell count that does not decease after the initial few drops. Xanthochromia (red/yellow) suggests haemoglobin degradation products and is also suggestive of a recent subarachnoid haemorrhage. Once subarachnoid haemorrhage is confirmed digital subtraction angiography is performed to identify a potential bleeding point for intervention. About 15% of patients will not have an aneurysm on angiography.

The main differential diagnoses of a SAH are a sentinel headache, cerebral venous thrombosis, acute hypertensive crisis and bacterial or viral meningitis.

SAH is associated with a mortality rate of up to 50%. Complications include rebleeding, cerebral infarction, hydrocephalus, cardiac ischaemia and hypothalamic dysfunction.

 KEY POINTS

- Sudden onset of severe headache should trigger investigation to rule out subarachnoid haemorrhage.
- A sentinel headache often precedes a severe subarachnoid haemorrhage.

CASE 57: COUGH AND JOINT PAINS

History

A 29-year-old man presents with a cough and some mild aches in the hands, wrists and ankles. The symptoms have been present for 2 months and have increased slightly over that time. Six weeks before, he had some soreness of his eyes, which resolved in 1 week.

The cough has been non-productive. He had noticed some skin lesions on the edge of the hairline and around his nostrils. Previously he had been well apart from an appendicectomy at the age of 17 years.

He was born in Trinidad and came to the United Kingdom at the age of 4 years. His two brothers and parents are well. He does not smoke, is a teetotaller, and takes no recreational drugs. He works as a messenger and took regular exercise until the last few weeks.

Examination

There is no deformity of the joints and no evidence of any acute inflammation. In the respiratory and cardiovascular systems there are no abnormal findings. In the skin there are some slightly raised areas on the edge of the hairline posteriorly and at the ala nasae. They are a little lighter than the rest of the skin.

INVESTIGATIONS

		Normal
Haemoglobin	13.5 g/dL	13.0–17.0 g/dL
Mean corpuscular volume (MCV)	88 fL	80–99 fL
White cell count	8.5×10^9/L	$3.5–11.0 \times 10^9$/L
Platelets	264×10^9/L	$150–440 \times 10^9$/L
Erythrocyte sedimentation rate (ESR)	34 mm	<10 mm/h
Sodium	140 mmol/L	135–145 mmol/L
Potassium	4.0 mmol/L	3.5–5.0 mmol/L
Urea	3.6 mmol/L	2.5–6.7 mmol/L
Creatinine	74 μmol/L	70–120 μmol/L
Bilirubin	14 mmol/L	3–17 mmol/L
Alkaline phosphatase	84 IU/L	30–300 IU/L
Alanine aminotransferase	44 IU/L	5–35 IU/L
Calcium	2.69 mmol/L	2.12–2.65 mmol/L
Phosphate	1.20 mmol/L	0.8–1.45 mmol/L

The chest X-ray is shown in Figure 57.1.

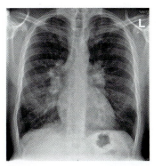

Figure 57.1 Chest X-ray.

Questions

- What is the likely diagnosis?
- How might this be confirmed?

ANSWER 57

The likely diagnosis is sarcoidosis. The age is typical, and sarcoidosis is more common in those of African-Caribbean origin. The chest X-ray shows bilateral hilar lymphadenopathy. The blood results show a slightly raised calcium level, which is related to vitamin D sensitivity in sarcoidosis, in which the granulomas hydroxylate 25-hydroxycholecalciferol to 1,25-dihydroxycholecalciferol. The ESR is raised, and some of the liver enzymes are around the upper limit of normal. The skin lesions at the hairline and the nostrils are typical sites for sarcoid skin problems. The eye trouble 6 weeks earlier might also have been a manifestation of sarcoidosis, which can cause both anterior and posterior uveitis.

An alternative diagnosis that might explain the findings is tuberculosis. Tuberculosis can also cause hypercalcaemia, although this is much less common than in sarcoidosis. Tumours, especially lymphoma, might give this X-ray appearance but would not explain the other findings. The arthralgia (pains with no evidence of acute inflammation or deformity on examination) can occur in sarcoidosis or tuberculosis, but again they are commoner in sarcoidosis. The ESR is non-specific. Arthralgia without deformity in an African-Caribbean man raises the possibility of systemic lupus erythematosus (SLE), but this would be much commoner in women and would not cause bilateral hilar lymphadenopathy.

He is likely to have had BCG (bacille Calmette–Guèrin) vaccination at school at around the age of 12 years, giving a degree of protection against tuberculosis. A tuberculin test should be positive after BCG, strongly positive in most cases of tuberculosis and negative in 80 per cent of cases of sarcoidosis. The serum level of angiotensin-converting enzyme would be raised in over 80 per cent of cases of sarcoidosis but often in tuberculosis also; the granuloma cells secrete this enzyme. A computed tomography (CT) scan of the chest will confirm the extent of the lymphadenopathy and show whether there is any involvement of the lung parenchyma. Histology of affected tissue would confirm the clinical diagnosis. This might be obtained by a skin biopsy of one of the lesions. A bronchial or transbronchial lung biopsy at fibre-optic bronchoscopy would be another means of obtaining diagnostic histology. In patients with a cough and sarcoidosis, the bronchial mucosa itself often looks abnormal, and biopsy will provide the diagnosis. Lung function tests and electrocardiogram (ECG) should be performed as a baseline if the diagnosis is confirmed.

Steroid treatment would not be necessary for the hilar lymphadenopathy alone but would be indicated for the hypercalcaemia and possibly for the systemic symptoms.

 KEY POINTS

- Sarcoidosis is commoner in those of African-Caribbean heritage.
- Typical sites for skin lesions are around the nose and the hairline.
- Sarcoidosis is a systemic disease and can affect most parts of the body.

CASE 58: THIRST AND FREQUENCY

History

A 63-year-old woman is referred to a nephrologist for investigation of polyuria. About 4 weeks ago she developed abrupt-onset extreme thirst and polyuria. She is getting up to pass urine five times a night. Over the past 3 months she has felt generally unwell and noted pain in her back. She has lost 3 kg in weight over this time. She also has a persistent frontal headache associated with early morning nausea. The headache is worsened by coughing or lying down. Eight years previously she had a left mastectomy and radiotherapy for carcinoma of the breast. She is a retired civil servant who is a non-smoker and drinks 10 units of alcohol per week. She is on no medication.

Examination

She is thin, and her muscles are wasted. Her pulse rate is 72/min, blood pressure is 120/84 mmHg, jugular venous pressure is not raised, heart sounds are normal, and she has no peripheral oedema. Examination of her respiratory, abdominal and neurological systems is normal. Her fundi show papilloedema.

INVESTIGATIONS		
		Normal
Haemoglobin	12.2 g/dL	11.7–15.7 g/dL
Mean corpuscular volume (MCV)	85 fL	80–99 fL
White cell count	6.7 × 10⁹/L	3.5–11.0 × 10⁹/L
Platelets	312 × 10⁹/L	150–440 × 10⁹/L
Sodium	142 mmol/L	135–145 mmol/L
Potassium	3.8 mmol/L	3.5–5.0 mmol/L
Bicarbonate	26 mmol/L	24–30 mmol/L
Urea	4.2 mmol/L	2.5–6.7 mmol/L
Creatinine	68 μmol/L	70–120 μmol/L
Glucose	4.2 mmol/L	4.0–6.0 mmol/L
Albumin	38 g/L	35–50 g/L
Calcium	2.75 mmol/L	2.12–2.65 mmol/L
Phosphate	1.2 mmol/L	0.8–1.45 mmol/L
Bilirubin	12 mmol/L	3–17 mmol/L
Alanine transaminase	35 IU/L	5–35 IU/L
Alkaline phosphatase	690 IU/L	30–300 IU/L

Urinalysis: no protein; no blood

Questions

- What is the likely cause of her polyuria?
- How would you investigate and manage this patient?

ANSWER 58

Polyuria is generally defined as a urine output >3litres a day in adults. True polyuria must be distinguished from frequency and nocturia which are generally due to bladder or prostate conditions.

This woman has mild hypercalcaemia, but this is not high enough to explain her extreme thirst and polyuria. It is more likely that she has polyuria due to neurogenic diabetes insipidus as a result of secondary metastases in her hypothalamus. The hypercalcaemia and raised alkaline phosphatase are suggestive of bony metastases secondary to her breast carcinoma. The recent-onset headache, worsened by coughing and lying down and associated with vomiting, is characteristic of raised intracranial pressure, which is confirmed by the presence of papilloedema. In some tumours around the pituitary there may be compression of the optic nerve, causing visual field abnormalities. Neurogenic diabetes insipidus is due to inadequate arginine vasopressin (AVP, antidiuretic hormone) secretion. About 30 per cent of cases of neurogenic diabetes insipidus are idiopathic. The remaining causes are neoplastic; infectious; inflammatory (granulomas); traumatic (neurosurgery, deceleration injury); or vascular (cerebral haemorrhage, infarction). Patients with central diabetes insipidus typically describe an abrupt onset of polyuria and polydipsia. This is because urinary concentration can be maintained fairly well until the number of AVP-secreting neurones in the hypothalamus decreases to 10–15 per cent of the normal number, after which AVP levels decrease to a range where urine output increases dramatically.

> **! Major causes of polyuria and polydipsia**
>
> - Solute diuresis (e.g. diabetes mellitus)
> - Renal diseases that impair urinary concentrating mechanisms (e.g. chronic renal failure), e.g. chronic renal failure.
> - Drinking abnormalities: psychogenic polydipsia
> - Renal resistance to the action of AVP
> - Nephrogenic diabetes insipidus (due to inherited defects in either the AVP V_2 receptor or the aquaporin-2 receptor)
> - Hypokalaemia
> - Hypercalcaemia
> - Drugs (e.g. lithium, demeclocycline)

A water-deprivation test should be performed in this patient, measuring the plasma sodium, urine volume and urine osmolality until the sodium rises above 146 mmol/L, or the urine osmolality reaches a plateau and the patient has lost at least 2 per cent of body weight. At this point AVP is measured, and the response to subcutaneous desmopressin is measured. An increase in urine osmolality >50 per cent indicates central diabetes insipidus and <10 per cent nephrogenic diabetes insipidus. The hypothalamus should be imaged by magnetic resonance imaging (MRI) scanning, and bone X-rays and bone scans should be performed to identify metastases (Figure 58.1). The MRI scan (T_1-weighted coronal image) through the pituitary in Figure 58.1 shows thickening of the pituitary stalk due to metastatic disease (short arrow) and partial replacement of the normal bone marrow of the clivus by metastatic tumour (long arrow). Treatment of the neurogenic diabetes insipidus involves regular intranasal DDAVP

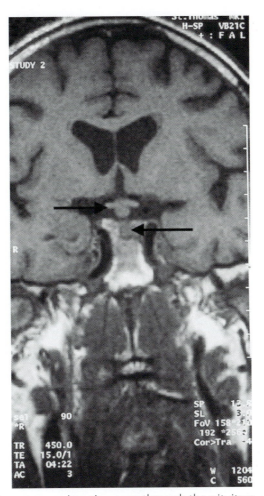

Figure 58.1 Magnetic resonance imaging scan through the pituitary.

(l-deamino-8-d-arginine vasopressin). She should be referred to an oncologist for treatment of her metastatic carcinoma.

 KEY POINTS

- The commonest causes of polyuria are diabetes mellitus and chronic renal failure.
- True polyuria must be distinguished from frequency and nocturia due to lower urinary tract pathology.
- Breast carcinoma may recur after several years of remission.

CASE 59: BLOOD IN THE URINE

History

A 52-year-old businessman is referred to a nephrologist for investigation of microscopic hae-maturia. This was first detected 6 months ago at an insurance medical for a new job and has since been confirmed on two occasions by his general practitioner (GP). His blood pressure was mildly elevated as his last medical exam. Previous urinalyses have been normal. He has never had macroscopic haematuria and has no urinary symptoms. He is otherwise in excel-lent health. There is no significant past medical history. He has no symptoms of visual prob-lems or deafness. There is no family history of renal disease. He drinks 35 units of alcohol per week and smokes 30 cigarettes per day.

Examination

He is a fit-looking, well-nourished man. His pulse is 72/min; blood pressure is 146/102 mmHg. Otherwise, examination of his cardiovascular, respiratory, abdominal and neurological sys-tems is unremarkable. Fundoscopy reveals arteriovenous nipping.

INVESTIGATIONS		Normal
Haemoglobin	13.6 g/dL	13.3–17.7 g/dL
Mean corpuscular volume (MCV)	83 fL	80–99 fL
White cell count	4.2 × 10⁹/L	3.9–10.6 × 10⁹/L
Platelets	213 × 10⁹/L	150–440 × 10⁹/L
Sodium	138 mmol/L	135–145 mmol/L
Potassium	3.8 mmol/L	3.5–5.0 mmol/L
Urea	8.2 mmol/L	2.5–6.7 mmol/L
Creatinine	141 µmol/L	70–120 µmol/L
Albumin	38 g/L	35–50 g/L
Glucose	4.5 mmol/L	4.0–6.0 mmol/L
Bilirubin	13 mmol/L	3–17 mmol/L
Alanine transaminase	33 IU/L	5–35 IU/L
Alkaline phosphatase	72 IU/L	30–300 IU/L
Gamma-glutamyl transpeptidase	211 IU/L	11–51 IU/L

Urinalysis: ++ protein; ++ blood; >100 red cells
24-h urinary protein: 1.2 g; normal <200 mg/24 h
Electrocardiogram (ECG): left ventricular hypertrophy
Renal ultrasound: two normal-size kidneys

Questions

- What is the likely diagnosis?
- What further investigations would you organize?
- What advice would you give this patient?

ANSWER 59

Microscopic haematuria has many renal and urological causes (e.g. prostatic disease, stones), but the presence of significant proteinuria, hypertension and renal impairment suggest this man has some form of chronic glomerulonephritis. The high gamma-glutamyl transpeptidase level is compatible with liver disease related to his high alcohol intake. The recommended upper limit for men is 28 units per week.

> **!** **Commonest glomerular causes of microscopic haematuria**
>
> - Immunoglobulin A (IgA) nephropathy
> - Thin basement membrane disease
> - Alport's syndrome (predominantly affects males)

IgA nephropathy is the commonest glomerulonephritis in developed countries and is characterized by diffuse mesangial deposits of IgA. Patients often have episodes of macroscopic haematuria concurrent with upper respiratory tract infection. Most cases of IgA nephropathy are idiopathic, but it is also commonly associated with Henoch–Schönlein purpura and alcoholic cirrhosis. This man has IgA nephropathy in association with alcoholic liver disease. About 20 per cent of patients with IgA nephropathy will develop end-stage renal failure after 20 years of follow-up.

Thin basement membrane disease is a familial disorder that presents with isolated microscopic haematuria, minimal proteinuria and normal renal function that does not deteriorate. Electron microscopy shows diffuse thinning of the glomerular basement membranes (the width is usually 150–225 nm versus 300–400 nm in normal subjects). Alport's syndrome is a progressive form of glomerular disease associated with deafness and ocular abnormalities and is usually inherited as an X-linked dominant condition, so males are more seriously affected.

This patient should have a renal biopsy to reach a histological diagnosis. As the patient is over 50 years old, he should have urine cytology/prostate-specific antigen/cystoscopy performed to exclude concurrent bladder and prostatic lesions. He needs a liver ultrasound, and liver biopsy should be considered.

The patient should be advised to abstain from alcohol and needs to have his blood pressure controlled. He needs regular follow-up as he is at risk of progressing to dialysis or renal transplantation. The raised creatinine appears modest in terms of the actual figures, but as plasma/serum creatinine does not begin to rise until the glomerular filtration rate is reduced to 50 per cent of normal (irrespective of the patient's age), the raised creatinine in this case indicates a serious loss of renal function to approximately 40 per cent of normal. There is no convincing evidence for immunosuppression retarding the progression into renal failure in most patients with IgA nephropathy.

> **KEY POINTS**
>
> - Patients with isolated haematuria aged less than 50 years should be initially referred to a nephrologist.
> - Patients with isolated haematuria aged more than 50 years should be initially referred to a urologist for investigation to exclude bladder or prostatic disease.
> - Small elevations in serum/plasma creatinine indicate large loss in renal function.
> - Liver damage from high alcohol intake may occur with no obvious signs and symptoms.

CASE 60: WEIGHT LOSS

History

A 67-year-old man attends his general practitioner's (GP's) surgery. He says that he has lost 10 kg in weight over the last 4 months. This has been associated with a decrease in appetite and an increasing problem with vomiting. The vomiting has been productive of food eaten many hours previously. During the last month he has noticed some weakness, particularly in his legs, climbing hills and stairs.

He is a smoker of 20 cigarettes per day and drinks around 10 units of alcohol each week. There is no relevant family history. His past medical history consists of hypertension, which was treated for 2 years with beta-blockers. He stopped taking these 4 months ago.

Examination

He looks thin and unwell. His pulse is 82/min. His blood pressure is 148/86 mmHg. No abnormalities are found on examination of the cardiovascular and respiratory systems. There are no masses to feel in the abdomen and no tenderness, but a succussion splash is present.

INVESTIGATIONS

		Normal
Sodium	130 mmol/L	135–145 mmol/L
Potassium	3.0 mmol/L	3.5–5.0 mmol/L
Chloride	82 mmol/L	95–105 mmol/L
Bicarbonate	41 mmol/L	25–35 mmol/L
Urea	15.6 mmol/L	2.5–6.7 mmol/L
Creatinine	100 μmol/L	76–120 μmol/L
Calcium	2.38 mmol/L	2.12–2.65 mmol/L
Phosphate	1.16 mmol/L	0.8–1.45 mmol/L
Alkaline phosphatase	128 IU/L	30–300 IU/L
Alanine aminotransferase	32 IU/L	5–35 IU/L
Gamma-glutamyl transpeptidase	38 IU/L	11–51 IU/L

Full blood count: normal
Chest X-ray: clear

Questions

- What is the likely explanation for these findings?
- What is the most likely diagnosis?

ANSWER 60

The clinical picture suggests obstruction to outflow from the stomach. This would be compatible with vomiting of residual food some time after eating and the succussion splash from the retained fluid and food in the stomach. The biochemical results fit with this diagnosis. There is a rise in urea but not creatinine, suggesting a degree of dehydration. Sodium, chloride and hydrogen ions are lost in the vomited stomach contents. Loss of hydrochloric acid produces metabolic alkalosis. In compensation, hydrogen ions are retained by exchange for potassium in the kidney and across the cell membranes, leading to hypokalaemia, and carbonic acid dissociates to hydrogen ions and bicarbonate. The hypokalaemia indicates considerable loss of total body potassium, which is mostly in the skeletal muscle, and explains the patient's recent weakness.

The most likely cause would be a carcinoma of the stomach involving the pyloric antrum and producing obstruction to outflow. A chronic gastric ulcer in this area could produce the same picture from associated scarring, and gastroscopy and biopsy would be necessary to be sure of the diagnosis.

Gastroscopy may be difficult because of retained food in the stomach. In this case, after this was washed out a tumour was visible at the pylorus, causing almost complete obstruction of the outflow tract of the stomach. The next step would be a computed tomography (CT) scan of the abdomen to look for metastases in the liver and any suggestion of local spread of the tumour outside the stomach. If there is no evidence of extension or spread, or even to relieve obstruction, laparotomy and resection should be considered. Otherwise chemotherapy and surgical palliation are treatment options.

 KEY POINTS

- Vomiting food eaten a long time previously suggests gastric outlet obstruction.
- Mild-to-moderate dehydration tends to increase urea more than creatinine.
- Prolonged vomiting causes a typical picture of hypochloraemic metabolic alkalosis.
- Carcinoma of the stomach can present without abdominal pain or anaemia.

CASE 61: LOSS OF CONSCIOUSNESS

History

A 52-year-old man is brought to the emergency department by ambulance. His wife gives a history that, while standing at a bus stop, he fell to the ground, and she was unable to rouse him. His breathing seemed to stop for about 20 s. He then developed jerking movements affecting his arms and legs and lasting for about 2 min. She noticed that his face became blue, and that he was incontinent of urine. He started to recover consciousness after a few minutes, although he remains drowsy with a headache. The man has not complained of any symptoms prior to this episode. There is no significant past medical history. He is a taxi driver. He smokes 20 cigarettes per day and consumes about 3 pints of beer each night.

Examination

The man looks fit and well nourished. He is afebrile. There is some bleeding from his tongue. His pulse is 84/min and regular. His blood pressure is 136/84 mmHg. Examination of his heart, chest and abdomen is normal. There is no neck stiffness, and there are no focal neurological signs. Funduscopy is normal. His mini-mental test score is normal.

INVESTIGATIONS		
		Normal
Haemoglobin	15.6 g/dL	13.3–17.7 g/dL
Mean corpuscular volume (MCV)	85 fL	80–99 fL
White cell count	5.2×10^9/L	$3.9–10.6 \times 10^9$/L
Platelets	243×10^9/L	$150–440 \times 10^9$/L
Sodium	138 mmol/L	135–145 mmol/L
Potassium	4.8 mmol/L	3.5–5.0 mmol/L
Urea	6.2 mmol/L	2.5–6.7 mmol/L
Creatinine	76 µmol/L	70–120 µmol/L
Glucose	4.5 mmol/L	4.0–6.0 mmol/L
Calcium	2.25 mmol/L	2.12–2.65 mmol/L
Phosphate	1.2 mmol/L	0.8–1.45 mmol/L

Questions

- What are the differential diagnoses of this episode?
- How would you investigate and manage this patient?
- What implications does the diagnosis have for this man's livelihood?

ANSWER 61

This man has had an episode characterized by sudden onset loss of consciousness associated with the development of generalized convulsions. The principal differential diagnosis is between an epileptic seizure and a syncopal (fainting) attack. Syncope is a sudden loss of consciousness due to temporary failure of the cerebral circulation. Syncope is distinguished from a seizure principally by the circumstances in which the event occurs. For example, syncope usually occurs while standing, under situations of severe stress or in association with an arrhythmia. Sometimes a convulsion and urinary incontinence occur. Thus, neither of these is specific for an epileptic attack. The key is to establish the presence or absence of prodromal symptoms. Syncopal episodes are usually preceded by symptoms of dizziness and light-headedness. Other important neurological syndromes to exclude are transient ischaemic attacks, migraine, narcolepsy and hysterical convulsions. Transient ischaemic attacks are characterized by focal neurological signs and no loss of consciousness unless the vertebrobasilar territory is affected. The onset of migraine is gradual, and consciousness is rarely lost. In narcolepsy, episodes of uncontrollable sleep may occur, but convulsive movements are absent, and the patient can be wakened.

In this man's case the episode was witnessed by his wife, who gave a clear history of a grand mal (tonic–clonic) seizure. There may be warning symptoms, such as fear, or an abnormal feeling referred to some part of the body—often the epigastrium—before consciousness is lost. The muscles become tonically contracted, and the person will fall to the ground. The tongue may be bitten, and there is usually urinary incontinence. Due to spasm of the respiratory muscles, breathing ceases, and the subject becomes cyanosed. After this tonic phase, which can last up to a minute, the seizure passes into the clonic or convulsive phase. After the contractions end, the patient is stuporous, which lightens through a stage of confusion to normal consciousness. There is usually a postseizure headache and generalized muscular aches.

In adults, idiopathic epilepsy rarely begins after the age of 25 years. Blood tests should be performed to exclude metabolic causes, such as uraemia, hyponatraemia, hypoglycaemia and hypocalcaemia. Blood alcohol levels and gamma-glutamyltransferase levels should also be measured as markers of alcohol abuse. A computed tomography (CT) scan of the brain is needed to exclude a structural cause such as a brain tumour or cerebrovascular event. This man should be referred to a neurologist for further investigation, including an electroencephalogram (EEG). This is necessary as he will probably not be able to continue in his occupation as a taxi driver. Treatment with anticonvulsants for a single seizure is also controversial.

 KEY POINTS

- It is vital to get an eyewitness account of a transient neurological episode to make a diagnosis.
- New-onset epilepsy is rare in adults and should therefore be fully investigated to exclude an underlying cause.

CASE 62: MEMORY LOSS

History

An 85-year-old woman attends her GP with her daughter. Her daughter says she is becoming more forgetful. On two occasions she has left the gas on the hob. She leaves the house but then can't remember why she left. She has become lost and been returned home by the police. She used to be diligent with her finances but recently her daughter found piles of unpaid bills. Her mother admits she gets a bit muddled trying to add up the amounts. Her writing has deteriorated and she struggles to think of the correct words. Her daughter says her mother can remember events from her earlier life fairly well but her short-term memory has gotten worse in the last 12 months. There has been no change in mood or appetite. There have been no hallucinations or delusions. Her mother has had no significant past medical history and has rarely needed to see doctors.

Examination

The examination of nervous, cardiovascular, respiratory and abdominal systems is entirely normal. Fundoscopy is normal. Abbreviated mental test scoring is grossly subnormal (3 out of 10).

! **Mini-mental state questionnaire**

- What is the name of this place?
- Can you remember this address I will give to you, '42 West Street'?
- What is the time?
- What year is it?
- What is my occupation?
- How old are you?
- When is your birthday?
- What year did World War II start and end?
- Who is the name of the current monarch?
- Who was the previous prime minister?

Questions

- What is the diagnosis?
- What are the major differential diagnoses of this condition?
- How would you investigate and manage this patient?

ANSWER 62

The abbreviated mental test score is a screening test for cognitive impairment. The score of 3 out of 10 indicates severe impairment of cognitive function. A thirty-point mini-mental state examination (MMSE) was performed and confirmed severe cognitive impairment. In this patient the diagnosis is **dementia**, with gradual decline in a number of higher centre cognitive domains (language, orientation, calculation, memory).

Dementia needs to be distinguished from delirium and depression. Dementia is a progressive decline in mental ability affecting intellect, behaviour and personality. In delirium, patients are acutely confused, inattentive and often have visual hallucinations. Delirium is usually reversible once the underlying cause is addressed (commonly infection, dehydration, medication and constipation). Patients with dementia are particularly vulnerable to delirium. Depression may mimic dementia (pseudo-dementia), as it can cause severe retardation of cognitive, vocabulary and motor functions. Depressed patients may score poorly on the abbreviated mental state test if they are rushed. Pseudo-dementia from depression is reversible with anti-depressant therapy.

Dementia is a syndrome that can be caused by many diseases. The commonest cause of dementia is Alzheimer's disease (AD). Progressive neuronal damage in AD occurs due to the accumulation of beta amyloid peptide with the formation of amyloid plaques and neurofibrillary tangles. The cause is not known. AD often begins as subtle forgetfulness and progresses over time such that patients lose their short-term memory, vocabulary, orientation. Later, long-term memory maybe lost, with an inability to remember relatives' names or perform everyday tasks. In the latter stages of AD, patients may not attend to personal hygiene, diet or liquid intake. The average time of death from diagnosis is 7 years.

> **! Causes of dementia**
>
> - Alzheimer's disease
> - Multi-infarct dementia
> - As part of progressive neurological diseases (e.g. multiple sclerosis)
> - Normal-pressure hydrocephalus: dementia, ataxia, urinary incontinence
> - Neurosyphilis: general paralysis of the insane
> - Vitamin B12 deficiency
> - Intracranial tumours; subdural haematomas
> - Hypothyroidism
> - AIDS dementia

The investigations in this patient should include a full blood count, erythrocyte sedimentation rate, serum urea and electrolytes, serum calcium, thyroid function tests, liver function tests, venereal disease research laboratory (VDRL) test for syphilis, vitamin B_{12} and folic acid, HIV serology and computed tomography (CT) of the head. In AD, the CT scan is usually normal or shows cerebral atrophy. Detailed neurocognitive testing may be helpful to identify the cause of dementia and can be used to detect early disease.

Oral cholinesterase inhibitors (donepezil, rivastigmine, galantamine) are modestly effective in treating AD, and may delay the need for nursing home care. Memantidine is an N-methyl-D-aspartate antagonist, which alone or in combination with a cholinesterase inhibitor is

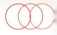

effective in moderate to severe AD. Special help is available in the UK for those caring for relatives with dementia. Help includes community occupational therapy, physiotherapy, community psychiatric team, an attendance allowance, respite care, daycare or lunch clubs, priority parking and carer support groups. Specialist memory clinics offer multi-disciplinary advice on treatment and support available.

KEY POINTS

- It is important to distinguish dementia from delirium and depression.
- Alzheimer's disease is the commonest cause of dementia.
- It may be possible to reverse or slow the progression of some types of dementia with specific treatments.

CASE 63: DIARRHOEA

History
A 35-year-old woman has a year-long history of intermittent diarrhoea, which has never been bad enough for her to seek medical help in the past. However, she has become much worse over 1 week, with episodes of bloody diarrhoea 10 times a day. She has had some crampy lower abdominal pain, which lasts for 1–2 h and is partially relieved by defaecation. Over the last 2–3 days she has become weak with the persistent diarrhoea, and her abdomen has become more painful and bloated over the last 24 h.

She has no relevant previous medical history. Up to 1 year ago, her bowels were regular. There is no disturbance of micturition or menstruation. In her family history, she thinks one of her maternal aunts may have had bowel problems. She has two children, aged 3 and 8 years, who are both well. She travelled to Spain on holiday 6 months ago but has not travelled elsewhere.

She smokes 10 cigarettes a day and drinks rarely. She took 2 days of amoxicillin after the diarrhoea began with no improvement or worsening of her bowels.

Examination
Her blood pressure is 108/66 mmHg. Her pulse rate is 110/min; respiratory rate is 18/min. Her abdomen is rather distended and tender generally, particularly in the left iliac fossa. Faint bowel sounds are audible. The abdominal X-ray shows a dilated colon with no faeces.

INVESTIGATIONS

		Normal
Haemoglobin	11.1 g/dL	11.7–15.7 g/dL
Mean corpuscular volume (MCV)	79 fL	80–99 fL
White cell count	8.8 × 10⁹/L	3.5–11.0 × 10⁹/L
Platelets	280 × 10⁹/L	150–440 × 10⁹/L
Sodium	139 mmol/L	135–145 mmol/L
Potassium	3.3 mmol/L	3.5–5.0 mmol/L
Urea	7.6 mmol/L	2.5–6.7 mmol/L
Creatinine	89 μmol/L	70–120 μmol/L

Questions
- What is your interpretation of these results?
- What is the likely diagnosis, and what should be the management?

ANSWER 63

Bloody diarrhoea 10 times a day suggests serious active colitis. In the absence of any recent foreign travel, it is most likely that this is an acute episode of ulcerative colitis on top of chronic involvement. The dilated colon suggests a diagnosis of toxic megacolon, which can rupture with potentially fatal consequences. Investigations such as sigmoidoscopy and colonoscopy may be dangerous in this acute situation and should be deferred until there has been reasonable improvement. The blood results show mild microcytic anaemia, suggesting chronic blood loss, low potassium from diarrhoea (explaining in part her weakness) and raised urea, but normal creatinine, from loss of water and electrolytes.

If the history was just the acute symptoms, then infective causes of diarrhoea would be higher in the differential diagnosis. Nevertheless, stool should be examined for ova, parasites and culture. Inflammatory bowel disorders have a familial incidence, but the patient's aunt has an unknown condition, and the relationship is not close enough to be helpful in diagnosis. Smoking is associated with Crohn's disease, but ulcerative colitis is more common in non-smokers.

Although amoxicillin treatment can be associated with bowel disturbance or even *Clostridium difficile* infection but it is not relevant here since the diarrhoea was present before taking amoxicillin and did not change afterwards.

She should be treated immediately with corticosteroids and intravenous fluid replacement, including potassium. If the colon is increasing in size or is initially larger than 5.5 cm in diameter, then a laparotomy should be considered to remove the colon to prevent perforation. If not, the steroids should be continued until the symptoms resolve, and diagnostic procedures such as colonoscopy and biopsy can be carried out safely. Sulphasalazine or mesalazine are used in the chronic maintenance treatment of ulcerative colitis after resolution of the acute attack.

In this case, the colon steadily enlarged despite fluid replacement and other appropriate treatment. She required surgery with a total colectomy and ileorectal anastomosis. The histology confirmed ulcerative colitis. The ileorectal anastomosis will be reviewed regularly; there is an increased risk of rectal carcinoma.

 KEY POINTS

- Bloody diarrhoea implies serious colonic pathology.
- It is important to monitor colonic dilatation carefully in colitis, and vital to operate before rupture.
- Both Crohn's disease and ulcerative colitis can cause a similar picture of active colitis.

CASE 64: PALPITATIONS

History

A 63-year-old man in police custody is brought to the emergency department because of palpitations. The palpitations are uncomfortable, rapid and began 2 hours ago whilst in the police station. He has had episodes of palpations in the past. He has no chest pain or dyspnoea.

He has a background of alcohol misuse and drinks 12 units of beer a day. He has type 2 diabetes mellitus, hypertension and asthma. He is not always adherent with his medications, which include metformin, gliclazide, ramipril, a salbutamol metered dose inhaler and a salmeterol with fluticasone metered dose inhaler.

Examination

He is conscious and smells of alcohol. His pulse is 185/minute and irregular, blood pressure is 126/73 mmHg and respiratory rate is 18 breaths per minute. Jugular venous pulse is not elevated. Heart sounds are normal with no added sounds. Breath sounds are normal with no added sounds.

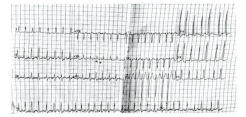

Questions

- What does the ECG show?
- What is the appropriate management of this patient?

ANSWER 64

The ECG shows atrial fibrillation (AF) evidenced by a narrow complex irregular tachycardia with no distinct p-waves. The previous episodes of palpitations are consistent with paroxysmal AF. The most likely cause for AF in this patient is hypertensive heart disease. Alcohol may be a trigger for atrial fibrillation. Other common causes include coronary artery disease and valvular heart disease. In younger patients conduction abnormalities such as Wolff–Parkinson–White (WPW) syndrome need to be considered. In WPW, a delta wave or short PR interval may be present on the ECG while the patient is in sinus rhythm. Atrial fibrillation can be secondary to a pulmonary embolism, hyperthyroidism, chronic lung disease and electrolyte abnormalities. Investigations should include measurement of electrolytes, thyroid function tests and a chest radiograph. An echocardiogram should be considered in this patient, as structural heart disease is common in older patients. If coronary artery disease is suspected then a cardiac stress test should be performed.

Atrial fibrillation can be classified as detected AF (first episode), paroxysmal AF (two or more episodes of AF) or persistent AF. Paroxysmal AF often evolves into persistent AF. In young patients without underlying structural heart disease the term 'lone AF' is used.

Atrial fibrillation is often asymptomatic. AF causes a reduction of cardiac output, which may result in hypotension and acute heart failure. Symptoms include palpitations, dizziness, dyspnoea and chest pain. AF also increases the risk of stroke. Thrombosis can form in the left atrial appendage and typically embolises to the cerebral arteries. Rarely, atrial thrombus can embolise to limbs or other organs. Persistent atrial fibrillation may cause structural changes to the heart muscle resulting in cardiomyopathy.

Acute management of atrial fibrillation should be resuscitation and control of heart rate. DC cardioversion may be required immediately if the patient is hypotensive or in acute pulmonary oedema. A beta blocker is recommended to control heart rate in those who are haemodynamically stable. Alternative agents include flecainide (if no underlying coronary heart disease), calcium channel blocker (if a beta blocker is contraindicated), or amiodarone or digoxin (useful if the patient has mild heart failure). Treatment should also be directed to any underlying cause of AF such as ischemic heart disease, hyperthyroidism or pulmonary embolism.

Long-term management of AF must include an assessment of thrombo-embolic risk and a decision regarding rate or rhythm control. The CHADS-2 score (see table 64.1) is used to calculate the risk of stroke associated with AF. Patients with a score of 1 or higher should receive long-term anticoagulation with warfarin. Newer anticoagulants, such as dabigatran, may be used as an alternative to warfarin. Unlike warfarin, dabigatran does not require regular monitoring of coagulation. Those patients with a contraindication to anti-coagulation should receive anti-platelet therapy such as aspirin or clopidogrel. Those patients with a CHADS-2 score of 0 can receive an antiplatelet or no treatment. Patients with paroxysmal AF should be assessed for stroke risk in the same way as those with persistent AF.

Table 64.1 CHADS-2 Score Stroke Risk[1]

Congestive cardiac Failure (+1)

Hypertension (+1)

Age >75 years (+1)

Diabetes (+1)

Prior TIA or stroke (+2)

Score 0 = 1.9% annual risk of stroke

Score 1 = 2.8% annual risk of stroke

Score 2 = 4.0% annual risk of stroke

Score 3 = 5.9% annual risk of stroke

Score 4 = 8.5% annual risk of stroke

Score 5 = 12.5% annual risk of stroke

Score 6 = 18.2% annual risk of stroke

(*Source:* Gage BF, van Walraven C, Pearce L, et al. Selecting patients with atrial fibrillation for anticoagulation: stroke risk stratification in patients taking aspirin. Circulation 2004:110 (16);2287–92. PMID 15477396.)

The decision to control rate or rhythm is based on the patient's age, length of time with AF and the presence of symptoms. There is no clear difference in mortality between a rate control or rhythm control strategy. Rate control aims to keep the heart rate under 100 beats per minute without the restoration of sinus rhythm. In general, a rate control strategy is used in older patients with longstanding and usually asymptomatic AF. A rhythm control strategy aims to restore and maintain sinus rhythm and is used in younger patients who have recent onset AF and experience symptoms. Restoring sinus rhythm can be achieved using medication (for example, amiodarone, sotalol, flecainide), elective DC cardioversion or by surgery. Surgery includes AV nodal ablation, pacing or pulmonary vein ablation.

In this patient, rate control was achieved with a calcium channel blocker, as a beta-blocker was contraindicated due to his asthma. Although his CHADS-2 score was two, warfarin was not recommended because of his history of alcohol misuse and poor medication adherence. Aspirin was prescribed to reduce his thrombo-embolic risk. A proton pump inhibitor was prescribed with the aspirin to prevent aspirin-induced peptic ulcer disease.

 KEY POINTS

- AF is often asymptomatic.
- AF is a risk factor for stroke. Patients at moderate or high risk for stroke (CHADS-2 score ≥1) should be anticoagulated unless there is a contraindication.
- Hypotension and acute pulmonary oedema as a result of AF are indications for immediate DC cardioversion.

History

A normally healthy man aged 28 years developed an acute sore throat, for which he consulted his general practitioner (GP). A diagnosis of acute pharyngitis was made, presumed streptococcal, and oral penicillin was prescribed. The sore throat gradually improved, but 5 days later the patient noted a rash on his arms, legs and face and painful ulceration of his lips and mouth. These symptoms rapidly worsened; he felt very unwell and presented to the emergency department. There was no relevant previous medical history or family history. He has had sore throats occasionally in the past, but they have resolved with throat sweets from the chemist.

Examination

He looked ill and had a temperature of 39.2°C. There were erythematous tender nodules on his arms, legs and face and ulcers with some necrosis of the lips and buccal and pharyngeal mucosae. The rest of the examination was normal.

INVESTIGATIONS

		Normal
Haemoglobin	13.8 g/dL	13.3–17.7 g/dL
White cell count	14.8 × 10⁹/L	3.9–10.6 × 10⁹/L
Platelets	334 × 10⁹/L	150–440 × 10⁹/L

Blood film: neutrophil leucocytosis

His chest X-ray is shown in Figure 65.1.

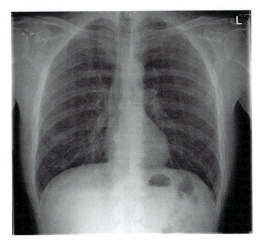

Figure 65.1 Chest X-ray.

Questions
- What is the diagnosis?
- What is the management?

ANSWER 65

The diagnosis is acute drug hypersensitivity causing severe erythema multiforme (Stevens–Johnson) syndrome. The pointers to this diagnosis are the rapidity of onset and its timing related to starting the penicillin, with antibiotics the commonest group of drugs causing this syndrome, and the form and distribution of the lesions. The chest X-ray shown is normal.

> **! Differential diagnoses of the rash**
>
> - Streptococcal (presumed) infection spreading to the soft tissues; this is much less common in young, healthy patients compared to the elderly; its distribution would be diffuse rather than discrete lesions and was excluded by negative culture of the lesions.
> - Acute leukaemia or neutropenia can present with mucosal ulceration, but not these skin lesions, and these diagnoses are excluded by the blood count and film.

Drugs other than penicillin (e.g. analgesics for the original painful throat) should be considered as a cause. The patient had taken a few doses of paracetamol, leaving the penicillin as the likeliest candidate by far as the cause.

> **! Management**
>
> Management consists of
>
> - stopping the penicillin and substituting an alternative antibiotic if required; cultures were negative in this case at this stage.
> - providing a short course of steroids (e.g. 30 mg prednisolone daily for 5 days to reduce the inflammation).
> - observing for secondary infection of the ulcers.
> - providing analgesia.
> - warning the patient not to take penicillin or related drugs in the future.
> - recording the penicillin allergy clearly in GP and hospital notes.

> **KEY POINTS**
>
> - A drug history is an essential part of every patient's history.
> - Always consider drugs as a cause of complications during a patient's illness.
> - Drug allergies should be recorded prominently in medical notes.

CASE 66: URINARY FREQUENCY

History
A 37-year-old man presents to his general practitioner (GP) with a 5-day story of urinary frequency, dysuria and urethral discharge. In the previous 24 h he had become unwell, feeling feverish and with a painful right knee. He works in an international bank and frequently travels to Asia and Australia, from where he had last returned 2 weeks ago. There is no relevant past or family history, and he takes no medication.

Examination
He looks unwell and has a temperature of 38.1°C. His heart rate is 90/min; blood pressure is 124/82 mmHg. Otherwise, examination of the cardiovascular, respiratory, abdominal and nervous systems is normal. His right knee is swollen and slightly tender, and there is a small effusion with slight limitation of flexion. There is no skin rash and no oral mucosal abnormality. He has a cream-coloured urethral discharge.

INVESTIGATIONS		Normal
Haemoglobin	17.1 g/dL	13.3–17.7 g/dL
White cell count	16.9 × 10⁹/L	3.9–10.6 × 10⁹/L
Platelets	222 × 10⁹/L	150–440 × 10⁹/L
Blood film: neutrophil leucocytosis		

His knee X-ray is shown in Figure 66.1.

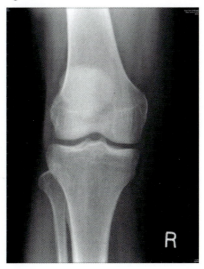

Figure 66.1 X-ray of the right knee.

Questions
- How would you investigate and manage this patient?
- What is the likely diagnosis?

ANSWER 66

The patient has acute gonorrhoea and gonococcal arthritis. The X-ray of the knee is normal. The diagnosis is made by microscopy of the discharge, which should show Gram-positive diplococci, and culture of a urethral swab. The swab should be inoculated to fresh appropriate medium straight away and kept at 37°C until arrival at the laboratory. Immediate treatment on clinical grounds with ciprofloxacin is indicated; penicillin should be reserved for gonorrhoea with known penicillin sensitivity to prevent the development of resistant strains. Septic monoarthritis is a complication of gonorrhoea; other metastatic infectious complications are skin lesions and, rarely, perihepatitis, bacterial endocarditis and meningitis.

The patient disclosed that he had had unprotected sexual intercourse with prostitutes in Thailand and Singapore; he had had no intercourse following return to the United Kingdom, so no follow-up of contacts was necessary. For advice on precautions and investigation for other sexually transmitted diseases he was referred to the sexually transmitted diseases (STD) clinic.

 KEY POINTS

- All students and doctors should be confident in eliciting a sexual history.
- Accurate sexual histories are more likely when the patient feels confidence and empathy with the interviewer.
- Contact tracing is an important element of management of sexually transmitted disease.

CASE 67: BACK PAIN

History

A 48-year-old woman presented to her general practitioner (GP) with a 3-month history of back pain in the midthoracic region. The pain was intermittent, worse at night, and relieved by ibuprofen, which she bought herself. She had no other symptoms and no relevant past or family history. She had never smoked and drank 10–12 units of alcohol most weeks. She worked part-time stacking the shelves in a supermarket and was a very active and competitive tennis and badminton player.

Examination

She looked well. She indicated that the pain was over the vertebrae at T5/6, but there was no tenderness, swelling or deformity. Her spinal movements were normal.

Her blood pressure was 136/76 mmHg. Cardiovascular, respiratory and abdomen examinations were normal.

 INVESTIGATIONS

Spinal X-ray was arranged and showed no abnormality. The full blood count, urea creatinine and electrolytes, calcium, alkaline phosphatase and phosphate were all normal, as was urine testing.

She was advised that the pain was musculoskeletal due to exertion at work and sport, and she was prescribed diclofenac for the pain. She was advised to rest from her tennis and badminton.

After a few weeks of improvement, the pain began to get worse, being more severe and occurring for longer periods and seriously disturbing her sleep. She returned to her GP and examination was as before except that there was now some tenderness over her midthoracic spine. The GP arranged another X-ray of the spine (Figure 67.1).

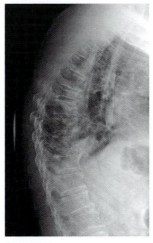

Figure 67.1 Lateral X-ray of the thoracic spine.

Questions
- What is the abnormality in the X-ray?
- What are the likeliest causes?

ANSWER 67

The X-ray shows collapse of the T6 vertebra. If there is nothing to suggest osteoporosis or trauma, then the commonest cause of this is a tumour metastasis. The tumours that most frequently metastasize to bone are carcinoma of the lung, prostate, thyroid, kidney, and breast. Examination of the patient's breasts, not done before the X-ray result, revealed a firm mass, 1- to 1.5-cm diameter, in the tail of the left breast. Urgent biopsy confirmed a carcinoma, and she was referred to an oncologist for further management.

The common lesions affecting the lumbosacral and cervical spine (e.g. inflammation of ligaments and other soft tissues and lesions of the intervertebral discs) are much less common in the thoracic spine, and bony metastases should be considered as a cause of persistent pain in the thoracic spine in patients of an appropriate age.

Review of the first X-ray after the lesion was seen on the second film still failed to identify a lesion, emphasizing the need to repeat an investigation if there is sufficient clinical suspicion of an abnormality, even if an earlier investigation is normal.

Examination of the breasts in women should be part of the routine examination, particularly after the age of 40 years, when carcinoma of the breast becomes common.

 KEY POINTS

- Pain in the thoracic vertebrae should raise the possibility of bony metastases in patients over the age of 40 years.
- Repeating previously normal or negative investigations is an important part of a patient's management when clinical diagnoses remain unconfirmed.

CASE 68: BREATHLESS ON EXERTION

History
A 59-year-old man attends his general practitioner because of exertional dyspnoea. In the last 12 months he has noticed that he is getting more breathless doing housework and walking up steps. He is also very fatigued. He has had no chest pain, cough or dizziness. He has no significant past medical history, but was told by a doctor years ago he had a heart murmur. He takes no medication. He has never smoked.

Examination
His pulse is 85/minute and regular, blood pressure is 128/73 mmHg and respiratory rate is 16 breaths per minute. He has a low volume carotid pulse and systolic thrill at the base of the heart. The apex beat is not displaced but is forceful. Second heart sound is soft and there is a harsh mid-systolic ejection murmur loudest over the second right intercostal space. The murmur radiates into the carotid arteries and is loudest during expiration. Breath sounds are normal with no added sounds. He has no peripheral oedema.

 INVESTIGATIONS

- Chest x-ray-shows cardiomegaly and normal lung fields.
- Electrocardiograph shows sinus rhythm and left ventricular hypertrophy.

Questions
- What is the murmur?
- How should this patient be managed?

ANSWER 68

The murmur is due to aortic stenosis. Typically aortic stenosis produces a murmur loudest in the aortic area that radiates to the carotid arteries. Its character is ejection systolic or crescendo-decrescendo. Left-side murmurs typically get louder with expiration as positive intrathoracic pressures increase the pressure difference across the valve (left-side murmurs loudest with expiration, right-side murmurs loudest with inspiration). The electrocardiogram shows left ventricular hypertrophy, which is a feature of aortic stenosis. Narrowing of the aortic valve causes left ventricular outflow obstruction. The left ventricle attempts to maintain cardiac output and hypertrophies in a response to an increased transvalvular pressure gradient created by the valve stenosis. Electrocardiograph and chest radiograph may show evidence of left ventricular hypertrophy. Causes of aortic stenosis include a congenitally abnormal valve with superimposed calcification, calcific disease of a previously normal aortic valve and rheumatic valve disease.

The presence of symptoms usually indicates the aortic stenosis is severe. Symptoms include exertional dyspnoea, fatigue, dizziness and chest pain. Approximately half of patients with aortic stenosis who present with chest pain have co-existing coronary artery disease. Signs of severe aortic stenosis include plateau pulse, an aortic thrill, length and lateness of the peak of the systolic murmur, 4th heart sound, paradoxical splitting of S2, absent A2 and signs of heart failure. An echocardiogram should be performed to assess the severity of the stenosis. Echocardiographic features of severe aortic stenosis include a valve area less than 1 cm² (normal 3–4 cm²), jet velocity over 4 m/s (normal <2.5m/sec) and a mean transvalvular pressure gradient exceeding 40 mmHg.

Aortic stenosis tends to progress over time and patients should be monitored with regular echocardiograms. The frequency of echocardiogram varies depending on the severity of AS; every 3 to 5 years for mild disease, 1 to 2 years for moderate disease and yearly for severe disease. Antibiotics before a dental or invasive procedure to prevent bacterial endocarditis are no longer recommended for patients with aortic stenosis. Patients with symptomatic and/or severe aortic stenosis should be referred to a cardiothoracic unit for aortic valve replacement. If valve replacement is not performed, the life expectancy is usually 2–3 years after the development of symptoms. This patient underwent an aortic valve replacement with resolution of his symptoms.

 KEY POINTS

- The development of symptoms in patients with aortic stenosis is an indication for aortic valve replacement.
- Aortic stenosis progresses over time and patients should be monitored with regular echocardiograms.

CASE 69: ABDOMINAL PAIN

History

A 58-year-old woman consults her general practitioner (GP); she has a 2-month history of intermittent dull central epigastric pain. It has no clear relationship to eating and no radiation. Her appetite is normal, she has no nausea or vomiting, and she has not lost weight. Her bowel habit is normal and unchanged. There is no relevant past or family history. She has never smoked and drinks alcohol very rarely. She has worked all her life as an infant school teacher. Physical examination at this time was normal, with a blood pressure of 128/72 mmHg. Investigations showed normal full blood count, urea, creatinine and electrolytes, and liver function tests.

An H_2 antagonist was prescribed and follow-up advised if her symptoms did not resolve. There was slight relief at first, but after 1 month the pain became more frequent and severe, and the patient noticed that it was relieved by sitting forward. It had also begun to radiate through to the back. Despite the progressive symptoms she and her husband went on a 2-week holiday to Scandinavia, which had been booked long before. During the second week her husband remarked that her eyes had become slightly yellow, and a few days later she noticed that her urine had become dark and her stools pale. On return from holiday she was referred to a gastroenterologist.

Examination

She was found to have yellow sclerae with a slight yellow tinge to the skin. There was no lymphadenopathy, and her back was normal. As before, her heart, chest and abdomen were normal.

INVESTIGATIONS		
		Normal
Haemoglobin	15.3 g/dL	11.7–15.7 g/dL
White cell count	6.2 × 10⁹/L	3.5–11.0 × 10⁹/L
Platelets	280 × 10⁹/L	150–440 × 10⁹/L
Sodium	140 mmol/L	135–145 mmol/L
Potassium	4.8 mmol/L	3.5–5.0 mmol/L
Urea	6.5 mmol/L	2.5–6.7 mmol/L
Creatinine	111 μmol/L	70–120 μmol/L
Calcium	2.44 mmol/L	2.12–2.65 mmol/L
Phosphate	1.19 mmol/L	0.8–1.45 mmol/L
Total bilirubin	97 mmol/L	3–17 mmol/L
Alkaline phosphatase	1007 IU/L	30–300 IU/L
Alanine aminotransferase	38 IU/L	5–35 IU/L
Gamma-glutamyl transpeptidase	499 IU/L	11–51 IU/L

Questions
- What is the likely diagnosis?
- What further investigations should be performed?

ANSWER 69

The patient has obstructive jaundice, as indicated by the history of dark urine and pale stools and the liver function tests. The pain has two typical features of carcinoma of the pancreas: relief by sitting forward and radiation to the back. An alternative diagnosis could be gallstones, but the pain is not typical.

As with obstruction of any part of the body, the objective is to define the site of obstruction and its cause. The initial investigation was an abdominal ultrasound, which showed a dilated intrahepatic biliary tree, common bile duct and gallbladder but no gallstones. The pancreas appeared normal, but it is not always sensitive to this examination owing to its depth within the body.

Further investigation of the region at the entrance of the common bile duct into the duodenum and head of the pancreas was indicated and was undertaken by computed tomography (CT) scan. It showed a small tumour in the head of the pancreas causing obstruction to the common bile duct, but no extension outside the pancreas. No abdominal lymphadenopathy was seen. No hepatic metastases were seen on this investigation or on the ultrasound. Alternative imaging techniques include magnetic resonance cholangiopancreatography (MRCP), which is used in preference to endoscopic retrograde cholangiopanreatography (ERCP) unless combined interventional procedures such as stone removal or stent insertion are also being considered.

The patient underwent partial pancreatectomy with anastomosis of the pancreatic duct to the duodenum. The jaundice was rapidly relieved. Follow-up is necessary not only to detect any recurrence but also to treat any possible development of diabetes.

 KEY POINTS

- Carcinoma of the pancreas can present with non-specific symptoms in its early stages.
- It is an important cause of obstructive jaundice.
- Patients who have had a partial removal of the pancreas are at risk of diabetes.

CASE 70: LEG WEAKNESS

History

A 24-year-old woman was attending her regular Sunday church service. During the singing of a hymn she suddenly fell to the ground without any loss of consciousness and told the other members of the congregation who rushed to her aid that she had complete paralysis of her left leg. She was unable to stand and was taken by ambulance to the emergency department. She has no other neurological symptoms and is otherwise healthy. She has no relevant past or family history, is on no medication, and has never smoked or drunk alcohol. She works as a sales assistant in a bookshop and until recently lived in a flat with a partner of 3 years' standing until they split up 4 weeks previously. She has moved back in with her parents.

Examination

She looks well and is in no distress, making light of her condition with the staff. The only abnormalities are in the nervous system. She is completely oriented and the Mini-Mental State score is normal. The cranial nerves and the neurology of the upper limbs and right leg are normal. The left leg is completely still during the examination, and the patient is unable to move it on request. Tone is normal; coordination could not be tested because of the paralysis. Superficial sensation was completely absent below the margin of the left buttock and the left groin, with a clear transition to normal above this circumference at the top of the left leg. Vibration and joint position sense were completely absent in the left leg. There was normal withdrawal of the leg to nociceptive stimuli such as firm stroking of the sole and increasing compression of the Achilles' tendon. The superficial reflexes and tendon reflexes were normal, and the plantar response was flexor.

Questions
- What is the diagnosis?
- How would you manage this case?

ANSWER 70

This patient has hysteria, now renamed dissociative disorder. The clues to this are the cluster of

- the bizarre complex of neurological symptoms and signs that do not fit neuroanatomical principles (e.g. the reflex responses and withdrawal to stimuli despite the paralysis)
- the patient's lack of concern, known by the French term of *la belle indifférence*
- the onset in relation to stress (i.e. the loss of her partner)
- secondary gain: removing herself from the parental home, which is a painful reminder of her splitting from her partner

None of these on its own is specific for the diagnosis, but put together they are typical. In any case of dissociative disorder, the diagnosis is one of exclusion; in this case the neurological examination excludes organic lesions. It is important to realize that this disorder is distinct from malingering and factitious disease. The condition is real to patients, and they must not be told that they are faking illness or wasting the time of staff.

The management is to explain the dissociation—in this case it is between her will to move her leg and its failure to respond—as being due to stress, and that there is no underlying serious disease such as multiple sclerosis. A very positive attitude that she will recover is essential, and it is important to reinforce this with appropriate physical treatment, in this case physiotherapy.

The prognosis in cases of recent onset is good, and this patient made a complete recovery in 8 days.

Dissociative disorder frequently presents with neurological symptoms, and the commonest of these are convulsions, blindness, pain and amnesia. Clearly some of these will require full neurological investigation to exclude organic disease.

 KEY POINTS

- Dissociative disorder frequently presents as a neurological illness.
- The diagnosis of dissociative disorder must be one of exclusion.

CASE 71: DROWSINESS

History

A 72-year-old woman develops a chest infection and is treated at home with doxycycline by her general practitioner (GP). She lives alone, but one of her daughters, a retired nurse, moves in to look after her. The patient has a long history of rheumatoid arthritis, which is still active and for which she has taken 7 mg of prednisolone daily for 9 years. She takes paracetamol occasionally for joint pain. There is no other relevant past or family history. When the GP visited he found her blood pressure to be 138/82 mmHg.

For 5 days she has been feverish and anorexic and confined to bed. Her daughter has made her drink plenty of fluids. On the fifth day she became drowsy, and her daughter had increasing difficulty in rousing her, so she called an ambulance to take her to the emergency department.

Examination

She is small (assessed as 50 kg), but there is no evidence of recent weight loss. Her temperature is 38.8°C. She is drowsy and responds to commands but will not answer simple questions. There is a global reduction in muscle tone but no focal neurological signs. Her pulse is 118/min, blood pressure is 104/68 mmHg, and the jugular venous pressure is not raised. There is no ankle swelling. In the chest there are bilateral basal crackles and wheezes. Her joints show slight active inflammation and deformity, in keeping with the history of rheumatoid arthritis.

INVESTIGATIONS		
		Normal
Haemoglobin	11.5 g/dL	11.7–15.7 g/dL
Mean corpuscular volume (MCV)	86 fL	80–99 fL
White cell count	13.2 × 10⁹/L	3.5–11.0 × 10⁹/L
Platelets	376 × 10⁹/L	150–440 × 10⁹/L
Sodium	125 mmol/L	135–145 mmol/L
Potassium	4.7 mmol/L	3.5–5.0 mmol/L
Urea	8.4 mmol/L	2.5–6.7 mmol/L
Creatinine	131 µmol/L	70–120 µmol/L
Glucose	4.8 mmol/L	4.0–6.0 mmol/L

Questions

- What is the diagnosis?
- How would you explain the abnormal investigations?
- How would you manage this case?

ANSWER 71

The likeliest diagnosis is secondary acute hypoaldosteronism due to failure of the hypothalamic–pituitary–adrenal axis caused by the long-term prednisolone use. This is a common problem in patients on long-term steroids and arises when there is a need for increased glucocorticoid output, most frequently seen in infections or trauma, including surgery, or when the patient has prolonged vomiting and therefore cannot take the oral steroid effectively. It presents as here with drowsiness and low blood pressure.

The hyponatraemia is another result of the superimposed illness. It is probably due to a combination of reduced intake of sodium owing to the anorexia and dilution of plasma by the fluid intake. In secondary hypoaldosteronism the renin–angiotensin–aldosterone system is intact and should operate to retain sodium. This is in contrast to acute primary hypoaldosteronism (Addisonian crisis), when the mineralocorticoid secretion fails as well as the glucocorticoid secretion, causing hyponatraemia and hyperkalaemia. Acute secondary hypoaldosteronism is often, but erroneously, called an Addisonian crisis.

Spread of the infection should also be considered, the prime sites being to the brain, with either meningitis or cerebral abscess, or locally to cause a pulmonary abscess or empyema. The patient has a degree of immunosuppression due to her age and the long-term steroid use. The dose of steroid is higher than may appear at first sight as the patient is only 50 kg; drug doses are usually denoted for a 70-kg male, which in this case would equate to 10 mg of prednisolone, that is, an increase of 40 per cent on her dose of 7 mg.

The treatment is immediate empirical intravenous infusion of hydrocortisone and saline. The patient responded, and in 5 h her consciousness level was normal, and her blood pressure had risen to 136/78 mmHg. Chest X-ray showed bilateral shadowing consistent with pneumonia, but no other abnormality.

 KEY POINTS

- Secondary hypoaldosteronism is a medical emergency and requires immediate empirical treatment.
- Patients on long-term steroids should have the dose increased when they have intercurrent illnesses and replaced systemically when they have persistent vomiting.

CASE 72: UNSTEADINESS

History

A 32-year-old woman presents to the emergency department with unsteadiness of gait for two days. The problem has been more evident at night but she feels a little unsteady on walking generally and on turning quickly. She had an upper respiratory infection a week or so earlier but has otherwise been well.

She smokes 10 cigarettes daily and drinks around 8–10 units of alcohol weekly. She has taken no recreational drugs. She is married with two children aged 2 and 6 years.

On systems review there are no problems with appetite, bowels, micturition, menses or any other symptoms.

Two years previously she had an episode of pain in the right eye associated with some blurring of vision in the right eye which lasted two to three weeks and then resolved spontaneously. She has had no subsequent visual problems. Her mother has type 2 diabetes mellitus.

Examination

She looks well. On neurological examination she has nystagmus on lateral gaze in both eyes. There is a mild degree of incoordination on heel–shin testing in the left leg. She is unsteady on heel–toe walking tending to fall to the left.

The blood pressure is 130/78 mmHg. On fundoscopy there is pallor of the right optic disc.

INVESTIGATIONS

		Normal
Haemoglobin	14.5 g/dL	11.7–15.7 g/dL
Mean corpuscular volume (MCV)	88 fL	80–99 fL
White cell count	8.2 × 10⁹/L	3.5–11.0 × 10⁹/L
Platelets	335 × 10⁹/L	150–440 × 10⁹/L
Sodium	137 mmol/L	135–145 mmol/L
Potassium	4.3 mmol/L	3.5–5.0 mmol/L
Glucose	7.1 mmol/L	4.0–6.0 mmol/L
Urea	4.7 mmol/L	2.5–6.7 mmol/L
Creatinine	84 µmol/L	70–120 µmol/L

Questions
- What is the most likely diagnosis?
- What further investigations would be appropriate?

ANSWER 72

The findings of unsteadiness, nystagmus and incoordination all point to a cerebellar problem producing her gait disturbance. The only abnormal investigation is slightly raised blood glucose. She has a family history of diabetes and her blood glucose warrants further testing, but it is unlikely to be related to her current problem.

In the previous medical history the episode of blurring of vision two years previously is characteristic of an episode of optic neuritis. Examination at the time would probably have shown a swollen pink optic nerve head. Residual changes may be the pale optic disc now and detailed testing might show a residual visual problem. Optic neuritis is associated with recurrence and progression to further demyelinating problems in about 50% of cases (greater in women than men).

The combination of these two problems indicates two neurological problems separated in space and time, in typical sites for demyelination and suggesting a likely underlying diagnosis of multiple sclerosis.

Further investigations should be magnetic resonance imaging to look for evidence of patchy demyelination. Abnormalities are found in the brain in over 90% of patients and in the spinal cord in about 75%. Oedema is shown on T2-weighted images and cerebral atrophy and areas of axonal death on T1 images. If a lumbar puncture is performed, cerebrospinal fluid should be sent for oligoclonal bands and intrathecal IgG production. She also needs a detailed ophthalmological assessment. Other possible investigations are evoked potentials (visual, somatosensory or auditory) which may show subclinical lesions and help in the diagnosis by suggesting other areas of demyelination.

Immunomodulatory treatment with intravenous steroids, immunoglobulin or plasmapheresis may help in the initial episode and in affecting future progression. Disease modifying agents such as interferon beta help in relapsing cases of multiple sclerosis. Once the diagnosis is confirmed she will need careful counselling around the question of possible future progression. She may benefit from contact with the Multiple Sclerosis Patients' Association.

 KEY POINTS

- Episodes of optic neuritis may be the first manifestation of multiple sclerosis.
- MRI is the optimal imaging technique for suspected multiple sclerosis.

CASE 73: CHEST PAIN AND SHORTNESS OF BREATH

History

A 25-year-old female accountant complains of shortness of breath, cough and chest pain. The chest pain came on suddenly 6h previously when she was walking to work. It was a sharp pain in the right side of the chest. The pain was made worse by breathing. It settled over the next few hours, but there is still a mild ache in the right side on deep breathing. She felt a little short of breath for the first hour or two after the pain came on but now only feels this on stairs or walking quickly. She has had a dry cough throughout the 6h.

She smokes 15 cigarettes a day and drinks 10 units of alcohol a week. She uses marijuana occasionally. She is on no medication. Four years ago something very similar happened; she is not sure but thinks that the pain was on the left side of the chest on that occasion. There is no relevant family history.

Examination

She is not distressed or cyanosed. Her pulse is 88/min, and blood pressure is 128/78 mmHg; respiratory rate is 20/min. Heart sounds are normal. In the respiratory system the trachea and apex beat are not displaced. Expansion seems normal, as is percussion. There is decreased tactile vocal fremitus, and the intensity of the breath sounds is reduced over the right side of the chest. There are no added sounds on auscultation.

🔍 **INVESTIGATIONS**

The chest X-ray is shown in Figure 73.1.

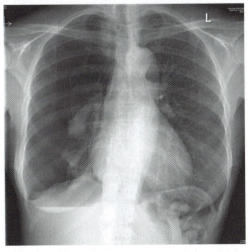

Figure 73.1 Chest X-ray.

Questions

- What does the X-ray show?
- What should be done now?

ANSWER 73

The chest X-ray shows a large right pneumothorax. There is a suggestion of a bullous lesion at the apex of the right lung. Pneumothoraces are usually visible on normal inspiratory films, but an expiratory film may help when there is doubt. There is no mediastinal displacement on examination or X-ray; movement of the mediastinum away from the side of the pneumothorax would suggest a tension pneumothorax. Although she had symptoms initially, these have settled down as might be expected in a fit patient with no underlying lung disease. A rim of air greater than 2 cm around the lung on the X-ray indicates at least a moderate pneumothorax because of the three-dimensional structure of the lung within the thoracic cage represented on the two-dimensional X-ray.

The differential diagnosis of chest pain in a young woman includes pneumonia and pleurisy, pulmonary embolism and musculoskeletal problems. However, the clinical signs and X-ray leave no doubt about the diagnosis in this woman. Pneumothoraces are more common in tall, thin men; in smokers; and in those with underlying lung disease. Further investigations such as computed tomography (CT) scan are not indicated unless there is a suggestion of underlying lung disease.

There is a suggestion that she may have had a similar episode in the past, but it may have been on the left side. There is a tendency for recurrence of pneumothoraces, about 20 per cent after one event and 50 per cent after two. Because of this, pleurodesis should be considered after two pneumothoraces or for those whose occupations might be affected, such as professional divers or pilots.

The immediate management is to aspirate the pneumothorax through the second intercostal space anteriorly using a cannula of 16-French gauge or more, at least 3 cm long. Small pneumothoraces with no symptoms and no underlying lung disease can be left to absorb spontaneously, but this is quite a slow process. Up to 2500 mL can be aspirated at one time, stopping if it becomes difficult to aspirate or the patient coughs excessively. If the aspiration is unsuccessful or the pneumothorax recurs immediately, intercostal drainage to an underwater seal or valve may be indicated. Difficulties at this stage or a persistent air leak may require thoracic surgical intervention. This is considered earlier than it used to be since the adoption of less-invasive video-assisted techniques has become widespread. In this woman the apical bulla was associated with a persistent leak and required surgical intervention through video-assisted minimally invasive surgery.

She should be offered support to stop smoking since tobacco smoking increases the risk of recurrence of pneumothorax. Marijuana has been reported to be associated with bullous lung disease, and this patient should be advised to avoid it.

 KEY POINTS

- The patient should not be allowed to fly for at least 1 week after the pneumothorax has resolved with full expansion of the lung (2 weeks after a traumatic pneumothorax).
- The risk of recurrence will be reduced by stopping smoking.

CASE 74: CONFUSION

History

An 79-year-old man has been in a residential home for 3 years since his wife died. He was unable to look after himself at home because of some osteoarthritis in the hips limiting his mobility. Apart from his reduced mobility, which has restricted him to a few steps on a frame, and a rather irritable temper when he doesn't get his own way, he has had no problems in residential care.

However, he has become much more difficult over the last 36 h. He has accused the staff of assaulting him and stealing his money. He has been trying to get out of his bed and his chair, and this has resulted in a number of falls. On some occasions his speech has been difficult to understand. He has become incontinent of urine over the last 24 h. Prior to this he had only been incontinent on one or two occasions in the last 6 months.

The duty doctor is called to see him and finds that he is rather sleepy. When roused he seems frightened and verbally aggressive. He thinks that there is a conspiracy in the ward, and that the staff are having secret meetings and planning to harm him. He is disorientated in place and time although reluctant to try to answer these questions.

He is a non-smoker and drinks 1–2 units a month. On a routine blood test 8 years ago he was diagnosed with hypothyroidism, and thyroxine 100 mg daily is the only medication he is taking. The staff say that he has taken this regularly up to the last 36 h, and his records show that his thyroid function was normal when it was checked 6 months earlier.

The nursing staff say that he is now too difficult to manage in the residential home. They feel that he has dementia, and that the home is not an appropriate place for such patients.

Examination

There is nothing abnormal to find apart from a blood pressure of 178/102 mmHg and limitation of hip movement with pain and a little discomfort in the right loin.

INVESTIGATIONS

		Normal
Thyroxine	125 nmol/L	70–140 nmol/L
Thyroid-stimulating hormone	1.6 mU/L	0.3–6.0 mU/L
Blood glucose	6.2 mmol/L	4.0–6.0 mmol/L
Urine dipstick: – sugar, + protein, ++ blood		

Questions
- What is the likely diagnosis?
- How should the patient be managed?

ANSWER 74

This is the picture of delirium. The four key features that characterise dementia are disturbance of consciousness, no obvious preexisting dementia, confusion that develops acutely (over hours or days) and tends to fluctuate during the day, and evidence of a precipitating cause such as a serious medical condition, substance abuse or medication side effect.

In contrast the cognitive changes in Alzheimer's disease are insidious, progressive and occur over a much longer time frame.

Common causes of delirium are fluid and electrolyte disturbances, infections, drug or alcohol toxicity, withdrawal from alcohol and drugs, metabolic disorders (hypoglycaemia, hypercalcaemia, liver failure), low perfusion states (shock, heart failure) and postoperative states.

In this case, there is no record of any drugs except thyroxine, although this should be rechecked to rule out any analgesics or other agents that he might have had access to or that might not be regarded as important. The thyroid abnormality is not likely to be relevant. The lack of replacement for 2 days will not have a significant effect and the normal results 6 months earlier make this an unlikely cause of his current problem. The sugar is normal. The falls raise the possibility of trauma, and a subdural haematoma could present in this way. However, it seems that the falls were a secondary phenomenon. The most likely cause is that he has a urinary tract infection. There is blood and protein in the urine, he has become incontinent and he has some tenderness in the loin which could fit with pyelonephritis. We are not told whether he had a fever, and the white cell count should be measured.

If this does seem the likely diagnosis it would be best to treat him where he is if this is safe and possible. He is likely to be more confused by a move to a new environment in hospital. There is every likelihood that he will return to his previous state if the urinary tract infection is confirmed and treated appropriately, although this may take longer than the response in temperature and white cell count. Treatment should be started on the presumption of a urinary tract infection while the diagnosis is confirmed by microscopy and culture of the urine. The most likely organism is *Escherichia coli*, and an antibiotic such as trimethoprim would be appropriate, although resistance is possible, and advice of the local microbiologist may be helpful. From the confusion point of view he should be treated calmly, consistently and without confrontation. If medication is necessary, small doses of a neuroleptic such as haloperidol or olanzapine would be appropriate.

 KEY POINTS

- Acute changes in mental state need to be explained even in the elderly with baseline mental problems.
- In delirium, consciousness is clouded, disorientation is usual, and delusions may develop. The onset is acute. In dementia, there is an acquired global impairment of intellect, memory and personality, but consciousness is typically clear.

CASE 75: UNCONSCIOUS AT HOME

History

A 21-year-old man is brought in to hospital at 5 pm. He was found unconscious in his flat by his girlfriend. She had last seen him at 8 pm the evening before when they came home after Christmas shopping. When she came to see him the next afternoon, she found him unconscious on the bathroom floor. He had been well previously, with no known medical history. There was a family history of diabetes mellitus in his father and one of his two brothers.

His girlfriend said that he had shown no signs of unusual mood on the previous day. He had his end-of-term examinations in psychology coming up in 1 week and was anxious about these, but his studies seemed to be going well, and there had been no problems with previous examinations.

He is a non-smoker. He drinks around 10 units of alcohol most weeks with occasional binges. He has taken ecstasy tablets in the past but has never used intravenous drugs.

Examination

He looks pale. There are no marks of recent intravenous injections. His pulse is 92/min, blood pressure is 114/74 mmHg, and respiratory rate is 22/min. There are no abnormalities found in the cardiovascular or respiratory system. In the nervous system, there is no response to verbal commands. Appropriate withdrawal movements are made in response to pain. The reflexes are brisk and symmetrical; plantars are downgoing. The pupils are dilated but responsive to light. In the fundi, the optic discs appear swollen.

Questions
- What are the most likely diagnoses?
- What other investigations should be done immediately?

ANSWER 75

This young man has been brought in unconscious, having been well less than 24 h previously. The most likely diagnoses are related to drugs or a neurological event. The first part of the care should be to ensure that he is stable from a cardiac and respiratory point of view. His respiratory rate is a little high. Blood gases should be measured to monitor oxygenation and ensure that the carbon dioxide level is not high, suggesting hypoventilation.

The family history of diabetes raises the possibility that his problem is related to this. However, the speed of onset makes hyperglycaemic coma unlikely. One would expect a slower development with a history of thirst and polyuria over the last day or so. However, the blood sugar should certainly be checked. Hypoglycaemia comes on faster but would not occur as a new event in diabetes mellitus. It might occur as a manifestation of a rare condition such as an insulinoma. Other metabolic causes of coma, such as abnormal levels of sodium or calcium, should be checked.

A neurological problem such as a subarachnoid haemorrhage is possible as a sudden unexpected event in a young person. Where the level of consciousness is so affected, some localizing signs or subhyaloid haemorrhage in the fundi might be expected. If no other cause is evident from the initial investigations, a computed tomography (CT) scan might be indicated.

The most likely cause is that the loss of consciousness is drug related. Despite the lack of any warning of intent beforehand, drug overdose is common, and the question of availability of any medication should be explored further. This would be likely to be a sedative drug. If there is any suspicion of this, then levels of other drugs that might need treatment should be measured (e.g. aspirin and paracetamol).

The other possibility in somebody brought in unconscious is that they are suffering from carbon monoxide poisoning. The fact that it is winter and he was found in the bathroom where a faulty gas-fired heater might be situated increases this possibility. Patients with carbon monoxide poisoning are usually pale rather than the traditional cherry-red colour associated with carboxyhaemoglobin. Papilloedema can occur in severe carbon monoxide poisoning and might account for the swollen appearance of the optic discs on funduscopy.

Measurement of carboxyhaemoglobin showed a level of 32 per cent. He was treated with high levels of inspired oxygen and made a slow but full recovery over the next 48 h. Mannitol for cerebral oedema and hyperbaric oxygen are considerations in the management. The problem was traced to a faulty gas water heater that had not been serviced for 4 years.

 KEY POINTS

- Drug overdose is the commonest cause of unconsciousness in young people, but other diagnoses must always be considered.
- Carboxyhaemoglobin levels should be measured in patients found unconscious indoors or in vehicles and after known exposure to smoke.
- In carbon monoxide poisoning, marked hypoxia may be present in the absence of cyanosis.

CASE 76: HEADACHE

History

A 24-year-old man presents to an emergency department complaining of a severe headache. The headache started 24h previously and has rapidly become more intense. He describes the headache as generalized in his head. He has vomited twice and appears to be developing drowsiness and confusion. He finds bright lights uncomfortable. There is no significant previous medical history or history of allergy. He smokes 10 cigarettes per day and drinks 24 units of alcohol per week. He is not taking any medication currently. He is a graduate student doing an MA in psychology. He lives with his female partner, and they have two children, aged 3 and 4 years.

Examination

He looks flushed and unwell. His temperature is 39.2°C. He has stiffness on passive flexion of his neck. There is no rash. His sinuses are not tender, and his eardrums appear normal. His pulse rate is 120/min, and blood pressure is 98/74 mmHg. Examination of heart, chest and abdomen is normal. His consciousness level is decreased, but he is rousable to command; there are no focal neurological signs. His fundi are normal.

🔍 INVESTIGATIONS

		Normal
Haemoglobin	13.9 g/dL	13.7–17.7 g/dL
White cell count	17.4 × 10⁹/L	3.9–10.6 × 10⁹/L
Platelets	322 × 10⁹/L	150–440 × 10⁹/L
Sodium	131 mmol/L	135–145 mmol/L
Potassium	3.9 mmol/L	3.5–5.0 mmol/L
Urea	10.4 mmol/L	2.5–6.7 mmol/L
Creatinine	176 µmol/L	70–120 µmol/L
Glucose	5.4 mmol/L	4.0–6.0 mmol/L
Blood cultures	results awaited	

Chest X-ray: normal
Electrocardiogram (ECG): sinus tachycardia
Computed tomography (CT) of brain: normal

Lumbar puncture	Turbid cerebrospinal fluid (CSF)	
Leucocytes	>8000/mL	<5/mL
CSF protein	1.4 g/L	<0.4 g/L
CSF glucose	0.8 mmol/L	>70 per cent Plasma glucose

Gram stain: result awaited

Questions
- What is the diagnosis?
- What are the major differential diagnoses?
- How would you manage this patient?

ANSWER 76

This patient has bacterial meningitis. He has presented with sudden onset of severe headache, vomiting, confusion, photophobia and neck stiffness. The presence of hypotension, leucocytosis and renal impairment suggests acute bacterial infection rather than viral meningitis. The most likely causative bacteria are *Neisseria meningitidis*, *Haemophilus influenzae* and *Streptococcus pneumonia*. In patients in this age group *Streptococcus pneumonia* or *Neisseria meningitidis* are the most likely organisms. Meningococcal meningitis (*Neisseria meningitidis*) is usually associated with a generalized vasculitic rash.

The most severe headaches are experienced in meningitis, subarachnoid haemorrhage and classic migraine. Meningitis and subarachnoid haemorrhage present as single episodes of headaches. Meningitis usually presents over hours, whereas subarachnoid haemorrhage usually presents suddenly. Fundoscopy in patients with subarachnoid haemorrhage may show subhyaloid haemorrhage. Meningeal irritation can be seen in many acute febrile conditions, particularly in children. Local infections of the neck/spine may cause neck stiffness. Other meningitis types include viral, fungal, cryptococcal and tuberculous meningitis, which can be distinguished by analysis of the CSF.

When meningitis is suspected appropriate antibiotic treatment should be started even before the diagnosis is confirmed. In the absence of a history of significant penicillin allergy, the most common treatment would be intravenous ceftriaxone or cefotaxime.

Patients with no papilloedema or lateralizing neurological signs that suggest a space-occupying lesion should be lumbar punctured immediately (even before a CT scan is obtained). If there are localized neurological signs it is essential to perform a CT scan first to avoid the dangers of coning, which can occur when a lumbar puncture is performed in the presence of raised intracranial pressure.

The combination of >1000 neutrophils/mL CSF, a CSF glucose <40 per cent of the simultaneous blood level and a CSF protein of 1.4 g/L is strongly suggestive of bacterial meningitis. The Gram stain and culture will give the definitive diagnosis. In this case, the Gram stain demonstrated Gram-positive cocci consistent with *Streptococcus pneumonia* infection. Intravenous antibiotics must be started immediately. The patient must be nursed in a manner appropriate for the decreased consciousness level. Adequate analgesia with opiates should be given. The patient has mild hyponatraemia due to the syndrome of inappropriate antidiuretic hormone (ADH) secretion, and fluid losses should be treated with normal saline. Inotropes may be needed to treat hypotension.

The two children aged 3 and 4 years must be considered. It is not clear from the history who is looking after them. They should be examined, and if meningococcal meningitis is suspected or the organism is uncertain, they should be given prophylactic treatment with rifampicin and vaccinated against meningococcal meningitis.

 KEY POINTS

- Bacterial meningitis causes severe headache, neck stiffness, drowsiness and photophobia.
- The main differential diagnoses are subarachnoid haemorrhage and migraine.
- When bacterial meningitis is strongly suspected, antibiotic treatment should be started before bacteriological confirmation is available.

CASE 77: ABDOMINAL PAIN

History

A 70-year-old woman has been complaining of upper abdominal pain, which has increased over the last 3 days. It has been a general ache in the upper abdomen, and there have been some more severe waves of pain. She has vomited three times in the last 24 h. On two or three occasions in the past 5 years, she has had a more severe pain in the right upper abdomen. This has sometimes been associated with feeling as if she had a fever, and she was treated with antibiotics on one occasion. Her appetite is generally good, but she has been off her food over the last week. She has not lost any weight. There have been no urinary or bowel problems, but she does say that her urine may have been darker than usual for a few days, and she thinks the problem may be a urinary infection.

In her previous medical history she has had hypothyroidism and is on replacement thyroxine. She has annual blood tests to check on the dose; the last test was 3 months ago. She has had some episodes of chest pain on exercise once or twice a week for 6 months and has been given atenolol 50 mg daily and a glyceryl trinitrate spray to use sublingually as needed.

Examination

Her sclerae are yellow. Her pulse is 56/min and regular. Her blood pressure is 122/80 mmHg. There are no abnormalities in the cardiovascular system or respiratory system. She is tender in the right upper abdomen, and there is marked pain when feeling for the liver during inspiration. No masses are palpable in the abdomen. She is clinically euthyroid.

INVESTIGATIONS		
		Normal
Sodium	139 mmol/L	135–145 mmol/L
Potassium	4.1 mmol/L	3.5–5.0 mmol/L
Urea	6.4 mmol/L	2.5–6.7 mmol/L
Creatinine	110 μmol/L	70–120 μmol/L
Calcium	2.44 mmol/L	2.12–2.65 mmol/L
Phosphate	1.19 mmol/L	0.8–1.45 mmol/L
Total bilirubin	83 mmol/L	3–17 mmol/L
Alkaline phosphatase	840 IU/L	30–300 IU/L
Alanine aminotransferase	57 IU/L	5–35 IU/L
Gamma-glutamyl transpeptidase	434 IU/L	11–51 IU/L
Thyroid-stimulating hormone	2.3 mU/L	0.3–6.0 mU/L

Questions

- How do you interpret these findings?
- What is the appropriate management?

ANSWER 77

This woman has a 5-year history of intermittent upper abdominal pain. Her current pain has lasted longer than previous episodes, and on examination she is jaundiced. The acute pain on inspiration while palpating in the right upper quadrant is a positive Murphy's sign of inflammation of the gallbladder. The relative bradycardia in the presence of the acute illness is likely to be related to the beta-blocker therapy (atenolol) rather than hypothyroidism or any other problem. The dark urine would fit with increased conjugated bilirubin because of obstruction. The conjugated bilirubin is water soluble and excreted in the urine. Without conjugated bilirubin entering the bowel, one would expect pale stools.

Her investigations show a raised bilirubin. The alanine aminotransferase is slightly raised, but the main abnormalities in the liver enzymes are high values of alkaline phosphatase and gamma-glutamyl transpeptidase. This is the pattern of obstructive jaundice, which can be caused by mechanical obstruction by tumour or by gallstones or by adverse effects of some drugs (e.g. phenothiazines, flucloxacillin). The drugs she is taking are not likely causes of liver problems.

The previous episodes of pain and fever over the last 5 years are likely to have been cholecystitis secondary to gallstones. If the gallbladder were to be palpable on examination, this would suggest an alternative diagnosis of malignant obstruction since by this time these previous episodes of cholecystitis would usually have caused scarring and contraction of the gallbladder. To produce obstructive jaundice one or more of her gallstones must have moved out of the gallbladder and impacted in the common bile duct. Migration of gallstones from the gallbladder occurs in around 15 per cent of cases.

Her thyroid condition seems to be stable and not relevant to the current problem. Her angina is indicative of coronary artery disease and needs to be considered when treatment is being planned for her gallstones. An electrocardiogram (ECG) should be part of her management.

Only a minority of gallstones are radiopaque and visible on a plain radiograph, so the next investigation should be an ultrasound of the liver and biliary tract. Ultrasound will show dilation of the biliary tree but is not so reliable for identifying common bile duct stones. Magnetic resonance cholangiopancreatography (MRCP) will clarify the site and cause of the obstruction and endoscopic retrograde cholangiopancreatography (ERCP) is the best tool for this, allowing intervention by sphincterotomy with or without stone retrieval to remove clear stones obstructing the common bile duct.

 KEY POINTS

- Obstructive jaundice with a dilated, palpable gallbladder is likely to be caused by carcinoma at the head of the pancreas (Courvoisier's sign).
- Obstructive jaundice causes preferential elevation of alkaline phosphatase and gamma-glutamyl transpeptidase.
- When the main rise is in alanine aminotransferase, this indicates primarily hepatocellular damage.

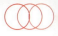

CASE 78: FEVER

History

A 36-year-old man presents to his general practitioner (GP) complaining of a fever and generalized aching in muscles around the back and legs. At first he thought that this was probably influenza, but the symptoms have now been present for 9 or 10 days. For 3 days he had diarrhoea, but this has settled now. He has complained of a sore mouth over the last week or so, which has made it difficult to eat, but he has not felt very hungry during this time and thinks he may have lost a few kilograms in weight. Around the time that the symptoms started, he noticed a mild erythematous rash over his chest and abdomen, but this has faded.

He has visited the practice occasionally in the past for minor complaints. He has been to the practice to obtain vaccinations for visits to Vietnam and Thailand over the last 3 years. His last travel abroad was 3 months ago. He smokes 10 cigarettes daily, drinks 20–30 units of alcohol weekly, and takes no illicit drugs. He has no other relevant medical or family history. He works as a solicitor. He is single and lives alone. He has had a number of heterosexual and homosexual relationships in the past. Twelve months ago he had an HIV test, which was negative.

Examination

He has a temperature of 38°C. Pulse rate is 94/min, respiratory rate is 16/min, and blood pressure is 124/78 mmHg. There are no abnormalities in the cardiovascular or respiratory system. On examination of the mouth, there are two ulcers in the oral mucosa, 5–10 mm in diameter. There are a number of palpable cervical lymph nodes on both sides of the neck, which are a little tender. There are no other nodes and no enlargement of liver or spleen. There are no rashes on the skin.

INVESTIGATIONS

		Normal
Haemoglobin	14.8 g/dL	13.7–17.7 g/dL
Mean corpuscular volume (MCV)	87 fL	80–99 fL
White cell count	7.4 × 10⁹/L	3.9–10.6 × 10⁹/L
Neutrophils	5.1 × 10⁹/L	1.8–7.7 × 10⁹/L
Lymphocytes	2.0 × 10⁹/L	0.6–4.8 × 10⁹/L
Platelets	332 × 10⁹/L	150–440 × 10⁹/L
Sodium	144 mmol/L	135–145 mmol/L
Potassium	4.4 mmol/L	3.5–5.0 mmol/L
Urea	5.9 mmol/L	2.5–6.7 mmol/L
Creatinine	73 µmol/L	70–120 µmol/L
Bilirubin	13 mmol/L	3–17 mmol/L
Alkaline phosphatase	121 IU/L	30–300 IU/L
Alanine aminotransferase	25 IU/L	5–35 IU/L

Screening test for glandular fever: negative

Question

- Can you suggest some possible diagnoses?

ANSWER 78

This seems likely to be an infective problem that has gone on for over a week. The length of the history makes influenza unlikely. The other positive features are the cervical lymphade-nopathy and the oral ulceration. The temperature is still up, and there has been a rash that has resolved. The blood results are all normal, including the test for glandular fever (infectious mononucleosis), which was a reasonable diagnosis with these features.

The previous homosexual contact increases the possibility of sexually transmitted infections. It is possible that travel to Vietnam and Thailand may have been associated with high-risk sexual exposure. He is known to have had a negative HIV test 12 months ago. However, it is quite possible that this might be an HIV seroconversion illness. In around half of those who acquire the virus, this occurs within 4–6 weeks of acquisition. Although the HIV test will still be negative, this can be diagnosed by finding the presence of the HIV virus or its p24 antigen in the blood. He should have been counselled about precautions to reduce the risk of transmission of sexually transmitted diseases at the time of the HIV testing 12 months before.

The picture might fit for secondary syphilis, which occurs 6–8 weeks after the primary lesion. However, in that case the rash would often be more extensive, and the lymph nodes are not usually tender. A serological test for syphilis should certainly be performed.

Other viral illnesses are possible. Hepatitis may present with this more general prodrome, but the normal liver function tests make this much less likely. Lymphoma can present with lymphadenopathy and fever, but the oral ulceration and the rash are not typical of lymphoma. If the serological tests proved negative, lymph node biopsy might be considered.

In this case, tests for an HIV viraemia were positive. Antiretroviral treatment at the time of known or high-risk exposure is useful in reducing the risk of infection. At this stage, treatment is supportive, with explanation and arrangements for monitoring of viral load.

 KEY POINTS

- A seroconversion illness occurs in around 50 per cent of those acquiring HIV infection. The severity varies.
- In cases of known or high-risk exposure, such as needlestick injuries, an immediate course of antiretroviral treatment is often indicated. Immediate advice should be sought.

CASE 79: EXCESSIVE DAYTIME SLEEPINESS

History

A 57-year-old male taxi driver presents to his general practitioner (GP) with excessive day-time sleepiness. For the last 2 years he has had a tendency to fall asleep whilst he is reading, watching TV or sitting quietly. On two occasions he has fallen asleep whilst driving. The first occurred at a traffic light. He was woken by the beeping of a car behind him. He also fell asleep whilst driving on a motorway and drifted into other lane before waking. He sleeps for 8 hours at night. He has woken a few times gasping for air. His wife reports he is a loud snorer. On some occasions he stops breathing and she has felt the need to prod him for him to resume breathing. He takes rampiril and bendroflumethiazide for hypertension. Overnight oximetry is performed and shown in figure 79.1.

Examination

On examination his body mass index is 41 kg/m². His blood pressure is 168/98 mmHg. His oropharynx is crowded and red. Tonsils are normal sized. Cardiopulmonary examination is normal.

INVESTIGATIONS

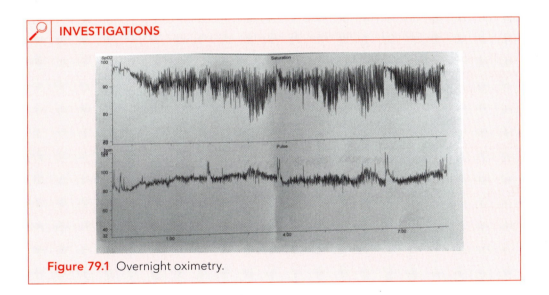

Figure 79.1 Overnight oximetry.

Questions

- What is the diagnosis?
- What is the management of this condition?
- What advice would you give him about driving?

ANSWER 79

The causes of excessive daytime sleepiness include inadequate sleep opportunity, obstructive sleep apnoea (OSA), narcolepsy, periodic limb movements in sleep, depression and medication. Despite adequate sleep opportunity (>7 hours) this patient describes excessive daytime sleepiness. This patient has symptoms of OSA with snoring, nocturnal dyspnea, witnessed apnoea and daytime sleepiness. Other symptoms of sleep apnoea include fatigue, poor concentration, nocturia, nocturnal choking, sore throat and morning headache. OSA is due to episodic collapse of the lumen of the upper airway during sleep. It results in airflow obstruction, oxygen desaturation and arousals from sleep. The frequent arousals from sleep result in daytime somnolence. Sleep apnoea causes hypertension and is a common cause of resistant hypertension. It is also an independent risk factor for heart disease and stroke. Patients may not be aware they have sleep apnoea and present with daytime sleepiness.

Sleep studies are required to confirm OSA. In this case, an overnight oximetry shows recurrent oxygen desaturations and heart rate rises consistent with OSA. Overnight oximetry is a useful tool; however, more detailed testing, such as an inpatient polysomnography, may be required if overnight oximetry is not diagnostic.

The treatment of sleep apnoea includes weight loss, mandibular advancement splints (MAS), and continuous positive airway pressure (CPAP). Tonsillectomy can be performed if tonsils are very enlarged, and is the commonest treatment of sleep apnoea in children.

CPAP is a device that provides positive airway pressure through a facemask. The positive pressure splints the upper airway open and prevents it from collapsing during sleep. CPAP is recommended for the treatment of moderate and severe OSA. Mandibular advancement splints are used in mild sleep apnoea. These are gum shields worn at night that pull the lower jaw forward and open the lumen of airway.

Obesity is a major reversible risk factor for OSA. The increasing prevalence of obesity worldwide has been accompanied by an increase in OSA. Weight loss should be recommended for all patients with OSA who are overweight (BMI ≥25 kg/m²). Dietary advice, behaviour modification and regular exercise should be recommended. Medication such as orlistat, which inhibits intestinal fat absorption, can also be also used. Bariatric surgery has a high success rate of weight loss and resolution of OSA. Bariatric surgery should be considered in patients with a BMI ≥40 kg/m² or BMI of 35 to 40 kg/m² with a co-morbid condition (such as diabetes mellitus, OSA or hypertension).

In most countries OSA is a notifiable condition to the driving authorities. In the UK this patient should not drive until treatment has started and sleepiness has resolved.

 KEY POINTS

- There is an increasing prevalence of obesity and OSA worldwide due to obesity.
- OSA presents with excessive daytime sleepiness and is a common cause of resistant hypertension.
- Treatment of OSA is usually with CPAP and weight loss.

CASE 80: PAIN IN THE CHEST

History

A 48-year-old man presents to the emergency department with discomfort in the left side of the chest. Ten days earlier he had felt unwell with a cough and some shortness of breath. He had also felt feverish. When these symptoms did not settle in 4–5 days he went to his general practitioner and was given some amoxicillin and paracetamol. After 48 hours he felt better and stopped taking the antibiotics.

Over the last two days he has been feeling unwell and has lost his appetite. He has also developed discomfort in the left side of the chest and has begun to feel feverish again. The cough has resolved but he is slightly short of breath on exertion.

There is no change in his bowels or micturition. He smokes 20 cigarettes per day and drinks 5 or 6 pints of beer most days. He is unemployed. His diet is poor and he has lost 6 kg in weight over the last year.

In his medical history he had an admission for a chest infection 6 years previously and has had treatment on and off for some years for peptic ulceration. There is no family history of note.

Examination

He is thin. His respiratory rate is 22/min, blood pressure is 124/76, pulse is 96/min, oxygen saturation is 95% breathing air. In the respiratory system there is some dullness to percussion with reduced breath sounds at the left base. X-ray is shown in Figure 80.1

INVESTIGATIONS		
		Normal
Haemoglobin	12.2 g/dL	11.7–15.7 g/dL
Mean corpuscular volume (MCV)	82 fL	80–99 fL
White cell count	18.9×10^9/L	$3.5–11.0 \times 10^9$/L
Platelets	450×10^9/L	$150–440 \times 10^9$/L
C-reactive protein (CRP)	282 mg/L	<5 mg/L

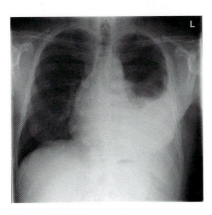

Figure 80.1 Patient's chest X-ray.

Questions

- What is the most likely diagnosis?
- How would you investigate and manage this patient?

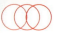

ANSWER 80

The sequence of the history suggests that this man had a partially treated pneumonia. The systemic symptoms, white cell count and inflammatory markers all indicate that there is a current problem with infection. The chest X-ray and the clinical findings show that there is a left pleural effusion. Pleural effusions can occur in association with pneumonia when they may be 'sympathetic' effusions related to the inflammation at the pleural surface of the lung. Such effusions resolve without further treatment as the pneumonia is treated. However, in this man it is more likely that the effusion is infected, i.e. an empyema. This needs to be established by aspiration of a sample of the fluid. This is best done under ultrasound guidance to reduce the likelihood of complications from the needle aspiration. This will also show whether there is one collection or loculation of the fluid as may occur with the intense inflammation associated with infection in the pleural space.

Empyemas are more likely to develop when there is inadequate antibiotic treatment or underlying problems with immunity. In this case antibiotics were discontinued too soon and his poor nutrition and high alcohol intake increase susceptibility.

In this case an ultrasound suggested some adhesions within the space but no distinct loculation. When a needle was inserted into the space, pus was aspirated. The pus had an overwhelmingly bad smell which permeated the side ward immediately. In this case it was obvious that the fluid was infected and the smell suggests that this is an anaerobic infection most commonly seen with the organism *Streptococcus milleri*. When the fluid is not obviously infected it should be sent for estimation of pH, protein, glucose and culture alongside a simultaneous blood glucose test. A pH <7.20 and low glucose are suggestive of infection in the pleural fluid.

As with any significant collection of pus empyemas require physical drainage as well as antibiotics. An adequate sized drain should be inserted, best placed under radiological control. If this fails to drain the fluid adequately thoracic surgical intervention may be required to break down adhesions or loculations and ensure adequate drainage. Thrombolytic agents have been used to help drainage but a meta-analysis suggested no significant benefit on outcome.

 KEY POINTS

- Pleural effusions associated with pneumonia may be sympathetic effusions or associated infection in the pleural space.
- Pleural aspiration and drainage should be done with ultrasound guidance.
- Adequate drainage for empyemas should be established as soon as possible after diagnosis.

CASE 81: ABDOMINAL PAIN

History

A 38-year-old man has a 2-month history of abdominal pain. The pain is epigastric or central and is intermittent. He had a similar episode a year before. On that occasion he took some indigestion mixture obtained from a retail pharmacy, and the symptoms resolved after 10 weeks. The pain usually lasts for 30–60 min. It often occurs at night, when it can wake him up, and seems to improve after meals. Some foods, such as curries and other spicy foods, seem to bring on the pain on occasions.

He has smoked 10–15 cigarettes per day for 25 years and drinks around 30 units of alcohol each week. He is not taking any medication at present. There is no other relevant medical history. He works as a financial broker in the city. He has been feeling more tired recently and had put this down to the pressure of work. A blood count was sent.

Examination

There is mild tenderness in the epigastrium, but no other abnormalities.

🔍 INVESTIGATIONS

		Normal
Haemoglobin	10.2 g/dL	13.3–17.7 g/dL
Red cell count	6.4×10^{12}/L	$4.4–5.9 \times 10^{12}$/L
Mean corpuscular volume (MCV)	71 fL	80–99 fL
White cell count	8.9×10^9/L	$3.9–10.6 \times 10^9$/L
Platelets	350×10^9/L	$150–440 \times 10^9$/L
Iron	4 mmol/L	14–31 mmol/L
Total iron-binding capacity	76 mmol/L	45–70 mmol/L
Ferritin	6 mg/L	20–300 mg/L

The blood film is reported as showing microcytic, hypochromic red cells.

Questions

- How do you interpret these findings?
- What is the likely diagnosis, and how should it be confirmed?

ANSWER 81

The blood count shows anaemia with a low MCV, indicating a microcytic anaemia. The high red cell count with low haemoglobin shows that the haemoglobin content of the cells is reduced. The low serum iron and ferritin with a high total iron-binding capacity (TIBC) confirm that this is related to true iron deficiency. The blood film confirms that the cells are microcytic and low in haemoglobin (hypochromasia). In anaemia of chronic disease the cells may be microcytic and serum iron low, but the TIBC would be low also and ferritin normal. The diagnosis is most likely to be a peptic ulcer.

The commonest cause of iron-deficiency anaemia in a man is gastrointestinal blood loss. In a premenopausal woman menstrual blood loss would be the commonest cause. The abdominal pains would be consistent with those from a peptic ulcer, especially a duodenal ulcer when there is more often some relief from food. The diagnosis should be established by endoscopy because alternative diagnoses such as carcinoma of the stomach cannot be ruled out from the history. The site of the blood loss causing the iron deficiency should be established. At the same time the presence of *Helicobacter pylori* should be investigated.

In this case, an endoscopy confirmed an active duodenal ulcer, and samples were positive for *Helicobacter pylori*. This is associated with gastritis and with over 90 per cent of duodenal ulcers. Tests of expired breath and serum antibodies are alternative diagnostic tests. The *H. pylori* was treated by a combined regimen of omeprazole for 6 weeks and triple therapy with lansoprazole, amoxicillin and clarithromycin for 7 days. For small (<1cm) uncomplicated ulcers there is no indication for continuing proton pump inhibitors after completion of the course of antibiotics. By contrast, continuing antisecretory therapy until the cure of *H. pylori* is confirmed is important for complicated ulcers. He was given strong recommendations to stop smoking and to address his excessive alcohol consumption. The importance of stress as a risk factor for peptic ulcer disease remains controversial. The iron deficiency was corrected by additional oral iron, which was continued for 3 months to replenish the iron stores in the bone marrow. Patients with uncomplicated duodenal ulcers who have been treated do not need further endoscopy unless symptoms persist.

 KEY POINTS

- Various antibiotic regimes have been shown to temporarily remove *Helicobacter pylori* and prevent or postpone recurrence of symptoms and ulceration.
- Replenishment of iron stores in the bone marrow needs 3 months of treatment with oral iron after the haemoglobin has returned to normal.
- Ferritin is an acute-phase protein and will be raised in the presence of acute illness even in the presence of iron deficiency.

CASE 82: ACHES AND PAINS

History

A 72-year-old woman has felt non-specifically unwell for about 10 weeks. She feels stiff, especially when she gets up in the morning. She struggles to get out of bed by herself. She has difficulty lifting her hand to comb her hair and has needed help with some of her housework. She has also noticed some pain in her knees and fingers. She has lost 4 kg in weight and has noticed some sweats, which seem to occur at night. She has come to see her general practitioner (GP) because she has now developed a headache. This is a severe pain that has been persistent over the last 4–5 days. On direct questioning she says that she has had some pain in her jaw when chewing. She has previously been fit with no significant past medical history. She lives alone. She has not smoked for 40 years, and she only drinks alcohol at Christmas. She is taking no regular medication. She has tried some paracetamol, but this has not helped the headache.

Examination

She is thin. She is tender to palpation over parts of her scalp. Her blood pressure is 138/64 mmHg. Examination of her cardiovascular, respiratory and abdominal systems is normal. Power is slightly reduced in the proximal muscles of her arms and legs (MRC scale 4+: active movement against gravity and strong resistance). Neurological examination is otherwise normal.

INVESTIGATIONS

		Normal
Haemoglobin	10.3 g/dL	11.7–15.7 g/dL
Mean corpuscular volume (MCV)	87 fL	80–99 fL
White cell count	12.2 × 10⁹/L	3.5–11.0 × 10⁹/L
Platelets	377 × 10⁹/L	150–440 × 10⁹/L
Erythrocyte sedimentation rate (ESR)	91 mm/h	<10 mm/h
Sodium	139 mmol/L	135–145 mmol/L
Potassium	4.6 mmol/L	3.5–5.0 mmol/L
Urea	3.8 mmol/L	2.5–6.7 mmol/L
Creatinine	102 μmol/L	70–120 μmol/L
Glucose	6.8 mmol/L	4.0–6.0 mmol/L
Albumin	38 g/L	35–50 g/L
Bilirubin	16 mmol/L	3–17 mmol/L
Alanine transaminase	85 IU/L	5–35 IU/L
Alkaline phosphatase	465 IU/L	30–300 IU/L
Creatine kinase	139 IU/L	25–195 IU/L

Questions

- What is the diagnosis?
- How would you investigate and manage this patient?

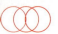

ANSWER 82

This woman has the typical clinical symptoms of polymyalgia rheumatica/giant cell arteritis. Most patients are over 65 years. The onset of symptoms is often sudden. Patients may present primarily with polymyalgia-type symptoms (proximal muscle pain and stiffness most marked in the mornings) or temporal arteritis symptoms (severe headaches with tenderness over the arteries involved). Patients may have systemic symptoms, such as general malaise, weight loss and night sweats. Characteristically, the ESR is very elevated (at least 40 mm/h), and there is a mild anaemia and leucocytosis. The liver enzymes are often slightly raised. In polymyalgia, the main symptoms are muscle stiffness and pain, which may simulate muscle weakness. The creatine kinase is normal, unlike in polymyositis.

The diagnosis of polymyalgia rheumatica is essentially a clinical diagnosis. A very elevated ESR is useful. Around 25 per cent of patients with giant cell arteritis have polymyalgia. When there are headaches and giant cell arteritis is suspected, a temporal artery biopsy should be performed. However, the histology may be normal because the vessel involvement with inflammation is patchy. Nevertheless, a positive result provides reassurance about the diagnosis and the need for long-term steroids.

This patient has clear evidence of giant cell arteritis (also known as temporal arteritis, although other vessels are involved) and is at risk of irreversible visual loss due to either ischaemic damage to the ciliary arteries causing optic neuritis or central retinal artery occlusion. The patient should immediately be started on high-dose prednisolone on the basis of the clinical picture before the biopsy is done. The results will not be affected by a few days of treatment and preservation of sight is the most important factor. The steroid dose should be slowly tapered according to clinical features and ESR but is likely to need to be continued for around 2 years. Bone protection measures should be part of the management.

! **Differential diagnoses of proximal muscle weakness and stiffness**

- Polymyositis
- Systemic vasculitis
- Systemic lupus erythematosus
- Parkinsonism
- Hypothyroidism/hyperthyroidism
- Osteomalacia

 KEY POINTS

- Polymyalgia rheumatica and giant cell arteritis often coexist.
- Patients with these conditions have markedly elevated ESR levels.
- There is a risk of blindness in giant cell arteritis, and steroids should be started immediately.

CASE 83: WEAKNESS

History

A 76-year-old woman presents to the emergency department complaining of an episode of weakness in her right arm and leg. She was sitting down with her husband when the weakness came on, and her husband noticed that she slurred her speech. All of the symptoms resolved within 10 min. Her husband has noticed two to three episodes of slurred speech lasting a few minutes over the last 6 months but had thought nothing of it. Two months earlier she had a sensation of darkness coming down over her left eye, lasting for a few minutes. She has had type 2 diabetes mellitus for 6 years, controlled on diet. She is hypertensive and suffered a myocardial infarction 3 years previously. She smokes about 10 cigarettes per day and drinks alcohol rarely. Her only medication is enalapril for her blood pressure.

Examination

She looks frail. Her pulse rate is 88/min and irregular, and blood pressure is 172/94 mmHg. The apex beat is displaced to the sixth intercostal space, midaxillary line. Her heart sounds are normal, and a grade 3/6 pansystolic murmur is audible. A soft bruit is audible on auscultation over the left carotid artery. Her dorsalis pedis pulses are not palpable bilaterally, and her posterior tibial is weak on the left and absent on the right. Examination of her chest and abdomen is normal. Neurological examination demonstrates normal tone, power and reflexes. There is no sensory loss. Funduscopy is normal.

🔍 INVESTIGATIONS

		Normal
Haemoglobin	13.7 g/dL	11.7–15.7 g/dL
Mean corpuscular volume (MCV)	86 fL	80–99 fL
White cell count	7.4×10^9/L	$3.5–11.0 \times 10^9$/L
Platelets	242×10^9/L	$150–440 \times 10^9$/L
Sodium	137 mmol/L	135–145 mmol/L
Potassium	3.9 mmol/L	3.5–5.0 mmol/L
Urea	6.7 mmol/L	2.5–6.7 mmol/L
Creatinine	86 µmol/L	70–120 µmol/L
Glucose	5.8 mmol/L	4.0–6.0 mmol/L
Haemoglobin A_{1c} (HbA$_{1c}$)	7.6 per cent	<7 per cent

Chest X-ray: normal
Electrocardiogram (ECG): atrial fibrillation

Questions
- What is the diagnosis?
- How would you manage this patient?

ANSWER 83

This woman gives a history of transient neurological symptoms with no residual signs. She is at increased risk of cerebrovascular disease because of her smoking, hypertension and diabetes. She is describing recurrent transient ischaemic attacks (TIAs), which by definition resolve completely in less than 24 h and, in practice, often much quicker. Two months before her admission she had an episode of amaurosis fugax (transient uniocular blindness) which is often described as like a shutter coming down over the visual field of one eye. The TIAs are affecting the left cerebral hemisphere in the area of brain supplied by the left carotid artery, causing right-sided weakness and dysarthria. TIAs may be caused by thromboembolism from ulcerated plaques in the carotid arteries or aortic arch, from cardiac sources such as a dilated left atrium, and more rarely due to haematological causes such as polycythaemia rubra vera, sickle cell disease or hyperviscosity due to myeloma. The symptoms may be the same each time or vary. Her ECG shows atrial fibrillation, and she has the signs of mitral regurgitation with a pansystolic murmur and displaced apex beat. There are three obvious potential sources for emboli:

- a left carotid artery stenosis (in a correct location to account for the distribution of these TIAs and more likely in the presence of a carotid bruit)
- the left atrium in atrial fibrillation with clinically evident mitral regurgitation
- a previous myocardial infarction with mural thrombosis.

! **Major causes of transient neurological syndromes**

- *Migraine*: the aura of migraine is a spreading and slowly intensifying phenomenon, and the symptoms are usually positive (e.g. scotomata). The aura is usually followed by a severe headache. However, migraines can be associated with focal neurological deficits (e.g. hemiplegia).
- *Focal epilepsy*: this also normally causes positive symptoms such as twitching and sensory symptoms, which may march up one limb and from one limb to another on the same side.
- *Syncope*: unlike most TIAs there is loss of consciousness, but there are usually no focal signs. Dizziness often precedes the attack.
- *Space-occupying lesion*: a cerebral tumour or abscess can produce fluctuating symptoms and signs. The symptoms are usually more gradual in onset and are often associated with headaches or personality changes.
- *Miscellaneous*: hysteria, cervical spondylosis, hypoglycaemia and cataplexy.

This patient should be investigated with computed tomography (CT) of the head to exclude a structural space-occupying lesion; echocardiography to assess left-atrial size, the mitral valve (to exclude infective valvular vegetations) and to rule out thrombus in the left ventricle related to the previous infarct; and a Doppler ultrasound of the carotid arteries. If a critical carotid stenosis (>70 per cent) is present, carotid endarterectomy should be considered. The patient should be anticoagulated with warfarin because of her atrial fibrillation and carotid stenosis. Her blood pressure and diabetes should be carefully controlled and her lipids measured and treated if appropriate.

KEY POINTS

- Most transient ischaemic attacks persist for only a few minutes.
- Approximately 40 per cent of patients with cerebral infarction have a prior history of transient ischaemic attacks.
- Multiple risk factors need to be taken into account in the investigation and management of vascular disease.

CASE 84: VOMITING

History

A 52-year-old man presents to the emergency department at 2 am vomiting fresh red blood. He is continuing to vomit large amounts of blood. He has no associated abdominal pain. His stools have been dark black for 48 hours.

He has a history of hypertension for which he takes atenolol. He drinks a bottle of wine a day.

Examination

He is anaemic and mildly jaundiced. There are spider naevi on his upper trunk. His pulse rate is 72/min and the blood pressure 94/55 mmHg lying down, dropping to 72/42 on standing. The spleen is palpable at 4 cm below the costal margin.

🔍 **INVESTIGATIONS**		
		Normal
Haemoglobin	6.7 g/dL	13.3–17.7 g/dL
Mean corpuscular volume (MCV)	81 fL	80–99 fL
White cell count	8.6 × 10⁹/L	3.9–10.6 × 10⁹/L
Platelets	39 × 10⁹/L	150–440 × 10⁹/L
Sodium	138 mmol/L	135–145 mmol/L
Potassium	3.9 mmol/L	3.5–5.0 mmol/L
Chloride	99 mmol/L	95–105 mmol/L
Urea	5.8 mmol/L	2.5–6.7 mmol/L
Creatinine	70 μmol/L	70–120 μmol/L
Bilirubin	67 mmol/L	3–17 mmol/L
Alkaline phosphatase	344 IU/L	30–300 IU/L
Alanine aminotransferase	64 IU/L	5–35 IU/L
Gamma-glutamyl transpeptidase	467 IU/L	11–51 IU/L

Questions

- What is the likely diagnosis?
- What is the appropriate management?

ANSWER 84

The most likely diagnosis is a variceal bleed due to underlying chronic liver disease secondary to alcohol. He has signs of chronic liver disease and his liver function tests are consistent with this. Other causes of upper gastrointestinal bleeding in patients with liver disease include peptic ulcer disease, Mallory–Weiss tear, portal hypertensive gastropathy and gastric antral vascular ectasia. Thrombocytopenia is common in cirrhosis due to a combination of reduced thrombopoietin levels, splenic sequestration of platelets and bone marrow suppression.

The estimation of blood loss is often difficult from a patient's story. Haematemesis is a frightening symptom and the amount may be overestimated. The haemoglobin level in this case is low and there is significant postural hypotension. His pulse is not fast as he is taking a beta blocker. He has signs of chronic liver disease. This is likely to be a very serious bleed. Only 50% of patients with varcieal haemorrhage stop bleeding spontaneously, and there is a very high risk of bleeding in the next 6 weeks.

The patient needs to be resuscitated with transfusion via a large-bore peripheral intravenous line or a central line. FFP and platelets are needed to correct coagulopathy and thrombocytopenia, respectively. Intravenous antibiotics reduce infectious complications in hospitalised cirrhotic patients.

Endoscopy is required to identify the bleeding point. Bleeding oesophageal varices should be treated with oesophageal band ligation or sclerotherapy. Balloon tamponade is effective at achieving short-term haemostasis, and may be used until more definitive treatment is available. Terlipressin or octreotide reduce bleeding. Transjugular intrahepatic portosystemic shunts or surgery are reserved for patients who continue to bleed despite the above measures.

After he has been stabilised he needs to be asked questions about his alcohol intake. He should be advised to abstain from alcohol. CAGE criteria consist of four questions and are commonly used as a screen for alcoholism:

- Have you felt the need to **C**ut down drinking?
- Have you ever felt **A**nnoyed by criticism of drinking?
- Have you had **G**uilty feelings about drinking?
- Did you ever take a morning **E**ye opener?

 KEY POINTS

- Acute variceal bleeds are less likely to stop spontaneously than other upper gastrointestinal haemorrhages.
- The CAGE questionnaire is useful as a screening tool for alcoholism.
- In some surveys alcohol is linked directly to around 25% of acute medical admissions.

CASE 85: TIREDNESS AND IRRITABILITY

History
A 33-year-old housewife has noticed that she is becoming tired and having difficulty coping with her two children, aged 6 and 4 years. She goes to see her general practitioner (GP) because she feels she may be suffering from anxiety and depression. She says that she has felt more irritable and anxious than usual. Her sleep is normal. Her appetite has been normal, but she has lost some weight. Her change in personality has been noticed by her husband and friends. She feels constantly restless and has difficulty concentrating on a subject for more than a few moments. Her increased anxiety has developed over the past 3 months. She has also noticed an increased frequency of bowel movements. Her periods have become lighter and shorter. She feels extremely tired and thinks that she has been prone to sweat more than usual. She has had no significant illnesses previously. She is a non-smoker and drinks 10 units of alcohol per week.

Examination
She appears agitated, and her hands are sweaty and tremulous. Her pulse is 104 and regular; her blood pressure is 130/70 mmHg. Her proximal muscles seem a little weak. There are no abnormalities in the cardiovascular, respiratory, abdominal or nervous systems. Investigations are organized by her GP.

INVESTIGATIONS

		Normal
Haemoglobin	13.3 g/dL	11.7–15.7 g/dL
White cell count	4.7×10^9/L	$3.5–11.0 \times 10^9$/L
Platelets	246×10^9/L	$150–440 \times 10^9$/L
Sodium	142 mmol/L	135–145 mmol/L
Potassium	4.6 mmol/L	3.5–5.0 mmol/L
Bicarbonate	22 mmol/L	24–30 mmol/L
Urea	5.2 mmol/L	2.5–6.7 mmol/L
Creatinine	78 µmol/L	70–120 µmol/L
Glucose	4.2 mmol/L	4.0–6.0 mmol/L

Urinalysis: no blood; no protein

Questions
- What is the most likely diagnosis?
- How would you manage this patient?

ANSWER 85

Although anxiety might produce some of these symptoms and signs, they fit much better with a diagnosis of hyperthyroidism. The neck should be examined carefully, and in this case there was a smooth goitre with no bruit over it. Blood tests showed a very low thyroxine-stimulating hormone (TSH) level and high free thyroxine (T4), confirming the diagnosis of hyperthyroidism due to a diffuse toxic goitre (Graves' disease). Hyperthyroidism may mimic an anxiety neurosis with marked restlessness, irritability and distraction. The most helpful discriminatory symptoms are weight loss despite a normal appetite and preference for cold weather. The most helpful signs are goitre, especially with a bruit audible over it, resting sinus tachycardia or atrial fibrillation, tremor and eye signs. Eye signs that may be present include lid retraction (sclera visible below the upper lid), lid lag, proptosis, oedema of the eyelids, congestion of the conjunctiva and ophthalmoplegia. Atypical presentations of thyrotoxicosis include atrial fibrillation in younger patients, unexplained weight loss, proximal myopathy or a toxic confusional state. The weakness here is suggestive of a proximal myopathy. The very low TSH level indicates a primary thyroid disease rather than the far less common overproduction of TSH by the anterior pituitary.

! Common causes of hyperthyroidism

- Diffuse toxic goitre (Graves' disease)
- Toxic nodular goitre
  - multinodular goitre (Plummer's disease)
  - solitary toxic adenoma
- Over-replacement with thyroxine

Blood should be sent for thyroid-stimulating immunoglobulin, which will be detected in patients with Graves' disease. Medical treatment for thyrotoxicosis involves the use of the antithyroid drugs such as carbimazole or propylthiouracil. These are given for 12–18 months, but there is a 50 per cent chance of disease recurrence on stopping the drugs. If this happens, radioiodine or surgery is indicated. Beta-blockers can be used to rapidly improve the symptoms of sympathetic overactivity (tachycardia, tremor) while waiting for the antithyroid drugs to act. Radioiodine is effective, but there is a high incidence of late hypothyroidism. Surgery is indicated if medical treatment fails or if the gland is large and compressing surrounding structures. In severe exophthalmos there is a risk of corneal damage, and ophthalmological advice should be sought. High-dose steroids, lateral tarsorrhaphy or orbital decompression may be needed.

  KEY POINTS

- Thyrotoxicosis may be difficult to differentiate from an anxiety state. In older patients, symptoms such as palpitations, breathlessness and oedema may predominate.
- The commonest causes of hyperthyroidism are Graves' disease or a toxic nodular goitre.

CASE 86: WEAKNESS OF THE LEGS

History

A 48-year-old man presents to the emergency department with weakness of his legs. Four weeks earlier he had an episode of gastroenteritis that lasted 4–5 days. Four days before admission he had a feeling that there was something wrong in his feet, and 3 days before admission he started to develop some difficulty in walking and this has progressed so that he now has difficulty standing. Both feet have also become painful over the last day or so. His bowels and bladder are functioning normally. He has no other significant medical history. He neither smokes nor drinks alcohol and is taking no medication. He in a local supermarket.

Examination

He looks well but is anxious. His pulse rate is 102/min, and blood pressure is 152/94 mmHg. His jugular venous pressure is not raised, and examination of his heart, respiratory and abdominal systems is otherwise normal. Neurological examination shows MRC grade 2/5 power below his knees and 3/5 power for hip flexion/extension. The tone in his legs is reduced. Knee and ankle reflex jerks are absent even with reinforcement. There is impaired pinprick sensation up to the knees and reduced joint position sense and vibration sense in the ankles. Neurological examination of his arms is normal.

🔍 INVESTIGATIONS

Initial haematology and biochemistry results are normal.
A lumbar puncture is performed with the following results:

		Normal
Cerebrospinal fluid (CSF): clear		
Pressure	170 mm CSF	<200 mm CSF
CSF protein	3.4 g/L	<0.4 g/L
CSF glucose	4 mmol/L	>70 per cent plasma glucose
Leucocytes	5/mL	<5/mL
Plasma glucose	4.5 mmol/L	4.0–6.0 mmol/L
Gram stain: no organisms		

Questions

- What is the diagnosis?
- What are the major differential diagnoses?
- How would you manage this patient?

ANSWER 86

The most marked feature in the history and examination is the loss of power. The reduced tone and absent reflexes indicate that this is a lower motor neuron lesion. The sensory disturbance is less severe, and he has a sensory level around L/3. This is the typical clinical picture of Guillain–Barré syndrome (acute idiopathic inflammatory polyneuropathy). This disorder is a polyneuropathy that develops usually over 2–3 weeks, but sometimes more rapidly. It most commonly follows *Campylobacter* gastroenteritis or a viral infection, and a fever is common. It predominantly causes a motor neuropathy, which can have a proximal, distal or generalized distribution. Distal paraesthesiae and sensory loss are common. Reflexes are lost early. Cranial and bulbar nerve paralysis may occur and respiratory muscle involvement can cause respiratory failure. The diagnosis is made from the clinical picture and can be confirmed with examination of the CSF and from nerve conduction studies. The CSF protein is usually raised, but the cell count is usually normal, although there may be mild lymphocytosis. The disorder is probably due to a cell-mediated delayed hypersensitivity reaction causing myelin to be stripped off the axons by mononuclear cells.

! Differential diagnoses of motor neuropathy

- Guillain–Barré syndrome
- Lead poisoning
- Diphtheria
- Charcot–Marie–Tooth disease (hereditary motor and sensory neuropathy)
- Poliomyelitis

An acute-onset neuropathy suggests

- Guillain–Barré syndrome
- porphyria
- malignancy
- some toxic neuropathies
- diphtheria
- botulism

This patient should be referred to a neurologist for further investigation and management. In this patient who presents with weakness and sensory signs, it is important to make sure there is no evidence of spinal cord compression or multiple sclerosis. However, these would tend to cause hypertonia, hyper-reflexia and a more distinct sensory level. His respiratory function should be monitored with daily bedside spirometry, and temporary non-invasive ventilator support or intubation may be necessary. Supportive care is the most important element of treatment. He should also be treated with either plasma exchange or intravenous immunoglobulin, which will speed up recovery. Most patients recover over a period of several weeks.

 KEY POINTS

- Guillain–Barré syndrome presents with predominantly a motor neuropathy, although sensory symptoms are usually present.
- There is often a history of an infective illness in the previous 3 weeks, often *Campylobacter jejuni.*

CASE 87: RECURRENT FALLS

History

An 85-year-old man is admitted to hospital because of a fall, in which he has sustained a mild facial laceration. In his history it becomes evident that he has had around eight falls over the last 3 months. He says that the falls have occurred in the morning on most occasions but have occasionally occurred in the afternoon. He does not think that he has lost consciousness, although he does remember a sensation of dizziness with the falls. He says that the falls have not been associated with any chest pain or palpitations. He does not remember tripping or any other mechanical trigger to the falls. He seems to return to normal within a few minutes of the fall. On two or three occasions he has hurt his knees on falling, and on one other occasion he hit his head. He lives alone, and there have been no witnesses to any of the falls.

He smokes five cigarettes a day and does not drink. He has an occasional cough with some white sputum, but he cannot remember whether he was coughing at the time of any of the falls. He was diagnosed as having hypertension at a routine well-man clinic 4 years ago and has been on treatment with a diuretic, bendrofluazide and doxazosin, for this. The blood pressure has been checked in the surgery on three or four occasions, and he was told that it has been well controlled. He was found to have a high fasting blood sugar 6 months before and had been advised to consume a diabetic diet. There is no relevant family history. He worked as a messenger until he retired at the age of 70 years.

Examination

He looks well. His pulse is 90/min and irregular. The blood pressure is 134/84 mmHg. The heart sounds are normal, and there is nothing abnormal to find on examination of the respiratory system or gastrointestinal system. There are no significant hypertensive changes in the fundi. In the nervous system, there is a little loss of sensation to light touch in the toes, but no other abnormalities.

INVESTIGATIONS		
		Normal
Haemoglobin	13.8 g/dL	13.7–17.7 g/dL
Mean corpuscular volume (MCV)	86 fL	80–99 fL
White cell count	6.9 × 10⁹/L	3.9–10.6 × 10⁹/L
Platelets	138 mmol/L	150–440 × 10⁹/L
Sodium	138 mmol/L	135–145 mmol/L
Potassium	4.2 mmol/L	3.5–5.0 mmol/L
Urea	4.6 mmol/L	2.5–6.7 mmol/L
Creatinine	69 µmol/L	70–120 µmol/L
Glucose (fasting)	6.5 mmol/L	4.0–6.0 mmol/L

Results of an electrocardiogram are shown in Fig. 87.1.

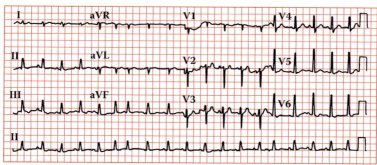

Figure 87.1 Electrocardiogram.

Question

- What are the most likely diagnoses?

ANSWER 87

There are a number of possibilities to explain falls in the elderly. Some more information in the history about the circumstances of these falls would be helpful. On further enquiry, it emerges that the falls are most likely to occur when he gets up from bed first thing in the morning. The afternoon events have occurred on getting up from a chair after his post-lunch doze. These circumstances suggest a possible diagnosis of postural hypotension. This was verified by measurements of standing and lying blood pressure—the diagnostic criteria are a drop of 15 mmHg on standing for 3 min. This showed a marked postural drop, with blood pressure decreasing from 134/84 to 104/68 mmHg. This is most likely to be caused by the antihypertensive treatment; both the alpha-blocker, which causes vasodilation, and the diuretic might contribute. Another possible candidate for a cause of the postural hypotension is the diabetes, which could be associated with autonomic neuropathy. In this case the diabetes is not known to have been present for long, and there is evidence of only very mild peripheral sensory neuropathy. Diabetic autonomic neuropathy is usually associated with quite severe peripheral sensory neuropathy, with or without motor neuropathy.

The electrocardiogram (ECG) shows evidence of sinoatrial node disease or sick sinus syndrome. Clinically, it is easily mistaken for atrial fibrillation because of the irregular rhythm and the variation in strength of beats. The ECG shows a P-wave with each QRS complex, although the P-waves change in shape and timing. It may be associated with episodes of bradycardia or tachycardia, which could cause falls. This might be investigated further with a 24-h ambulatory recording of the ECG.

Coughing bouts can cause falls through cough syncope. The positive intrathoracic pressure during coughing limits venous return to the heart. The cough is usually quite marked, and he might be expected to remember this since he gives a good account of the falls otherwise. Syncope can occur in association with micturition. Neck movements with vertebrobasilar disease, poor eyesight and problems with balance are other common causes of falls in the elderly. A neurological cause, such as transient ischaemic episodes and epilepsy, is less likely with the lack of prior symptoms and the swift recovery with clear consciousness and no neurological signs.

Another diagnosis that should be remembered in older people who fall is a subdural haematoma. Symptoms may fluctuate, and this might be considered and ruled out with a computed tomography (CT) scan of the brain.

The doxazosin should be stopped and another antihypertensive agent started if necessary. This might be a beta-blocker, long-acting calcium antagonist or angiotensin converting-enzyme (ACE) inhibitor, although all these can cause postural drops in blood pressure. His symptoms all disappeared on withdrawal of the doxazosin. The blood pressure rose to 144/86 mmHg lying and 142/84 mmHg standing, indicating no significant postural hypotension, with reasonable blood pressure control.

 KEY POINTS

- Falls in the elderly are a symptom in need of a diagnosis.
- Postural hypotension is a common side effect of diuretics, vasodilators or other antihypertensive therapy. Lying and standing blood pressures should be measured if this is suspected.
- Autonomic neuropathy in diabetes is associated with significant peripheral sensory neuropathy..

CASE 88: FATIGUE

History

A 63-year-old woman is brought in to the surgery by her neighbour, who has been worried that she looks increasingly unwell. On direct questioning she says that she has felt increasingly tired for around 2 years. She has been off her food but is unclear whether she has lost any weight. She was diagnosed with hypothyroidism 8 years ago and has been on thyroxine replacement but has not had her blood tests checked for a few years. Her other complaints are of itching for 2–3 months, but she has not noticed any rash. She says that her mouth has been dry and, on direct questioning, thinks her eyes have also felt dry.

There has been no disturbance of her bowels or urine, although she thinks that her urine has been rather 'strong' lately. She is 14 years postmenopausal. There is a family history of thyroid disease and of diabetes. She does not smoke and drinks two glasses of sherry every weekend. She has never drunk more than this regularly. She has taken occasional paracetamol for headaches but has been on no regular medication other than thyroxine and some vitamin tablets she buys from the chemist.

Examination

Her sclerae look a little yellow, and she has xanthelasmata around the eyes. There are some excoriated marks from scratching over her back and upper arms. The pulse is 74/min and regular; blood pressure is 128/76 mmHg. No abnormalities are found in the cardiovascular or respiratory system. In the abdomen, the liver is not palpable, but the spleen is felt 2 cm under the left costal margin. It is not tender.

INVESTIGATIONS		
		Normal
Sodium	142 mmol/L	135–145 mmol/L
Potassium	4.2 mmol/L	3.5–5.0 mmol/L
Urea	5.6 mmol/L	2.5–6.7 mmol/L
Creatinine	84 µmol/L	70–120 µmol/L
Calcium	2.24 mmol/L	2.12–2.65 mmol/L
Phosphate	1.09 mmol/L	0.8–1.45 mmol/L
Total bilirubin	84 mmol/L	3–17 mmol/L
Alkaline phosphatase	494 IU/L	30–300 IU/L
Alanine aminotransferase	63 IU/L	5–35 IU/L
Gamma-glutamyl transpeptidase	568 IU/L	11–51 IU/L
Thyroid-stimulating hormone	1.2 mU/L	0.3–6.0 mU/L
Cholesterol	7.8 mmol/L	<5.5 mmol/L
Fasting glucose	4.7 mmol/L	4.0–6.0 mmol/L

Antinuclear antibody: +
Antimitochondrial antibody: +++
Thyroid antibodies: ++

Questions

- What is your interpretation of these findings?
- What is the likely diagnosis, and how might this be confirmed?

ANSWER 88

The liver function tests show a predominantly obstructive picture with raised alkaline phosphatase and gamma-glutamyl transpeptidase, while cellular enzymes are only slightly raised. The symptoms (fatigue and pruritus) and investigations are characteristic of primary biliary cirrhosis, an uncommon condition found mainly in middle-aged women. In the liver there is chronic inflammation around the small bile ducts in the portal tracts. Fatigue is often a major factor that can impair quality of life. Itching occurs because of raised levels of bile salts, and can be helped by the use of a binding agent such as cholestyramine which interferes with their reabsorption. Hypercholesterolaemia, xanthelasmata and xanthomata are common. About 25–50 per cent of newly diagnosed patients have hyperpigmetation of the skin due to melanin deposition.The dry eyes and dry mouth may occur as part of an associated sicca syndrome. The presence of antimitochondrial antibodies in the blood is typical of primary biliary cirrhosis. These antibodies are found in 95 per cent of cases.

Hypothyroidism might explain some of her symptoms, but the normal thyroid-stimulating hormone (TSH) level shows that her current dose of 150 µg thyroxine is providing adequate replacement. The thyroid antibodies reflect the autoimmune thyroid disease, which is associated with other autoantibody-linked conditions, such as primary biliary cirrhosis.

The diagnosis is confirmed by a liver biopsy. This should be carried out only after an ultrasound confirms that there is no obstruction of larger bile ducts. Ultrasound will help to rule out other causes of obstructive jaundice, although the clinical picture described here is typical of primary biliary cirrhosis. No treatment is known to affect the clinical course of this condition.

 KEY POINTS

- The diagnosis of primary biliary cirrhosis should be considered in a patient complaining of unexplained itching, fatigue, jaundice or unexplained weight loss.
- Symptoms such as itching have a wide differential diagnosis. Dealing with the underlying cause, wherever possible, is preferable to symptomatic treatment.

CASE 89: LOSS OF CONSCIOUSNESS

History

A 40-year-old man is admitted to the emergency department having been found unconscious at home by his wife on her return from work in the evening. He has suffered from insulin-dependent diabetes mellitus for 24 years, and his diabetic control is poor. He has had recurrent hypoglycaemic episodes and has been treated in the emergency department on two occasions for this. Over the past few weeks he has developed pain in his right foot. His general practitioner diagnosed cellulitis, and he has received two courses of oral antibiotics. This has made him feel unwell, and he has complained to his wife of fatigue and anorexia and feeling thirsty. In his medical history he had a myocardial infarction 2 years ago. He has had bilateral laser treatment for proliferative diabetic retinopathy. He was a builder but is now unemployed. He smokes 25 cigarettes per week and drinks around 30 units of alcohol per week. His treatment is twice-daily insulin; he checks his blood glucose irregularly at home.

Examination

He is looks dry with reduced skin turgor and poor capillary return. His pulse is regular and 116/min. His blood pressure is 98/72 mmHg lying, 74/50 mmHg sitting up. He seems short of breath, with a respiratory rate of 30/min. Otherwise, examination of his respiratory and abdominal systems is normal. He has an ulcer on the third toe of his right foot, and the foot looks red and feels warm. He is rousable only to painful stimuli. There is no focal neurology. Funduscopy shows bilateral scars of laser therapy.

INVESTIGATIONS		
		Normal
Haemoglobin	15.2 g/dL	11.7–15.7 g/dL
White cell count	16.3 × 10⁹/L	3.5–11.0 × 10⁹/L
Platelets	344 × 10⁹/L	150–440 × 10⁹/L
Sodium	143 mmol/L	135–145 mmol/L
Potassium	5.5 mmol/L	3.5–5.0 mmol/L
Chloride	105 mmol/L	95–105 mmol/L
Urea	11.3 mmol/L	2.5–6.7 mmol/L
Creatinine	114 µmol/L	70–120 µmol/L
Bicarbonate	12 mmol/L	24–30 mmol/L
Urinalysis: ++ protein; ++ ketones; +++ glucose		
Blood gases on air		
pH	7.27	7.38–7.44
$PaCO_2$	3.0 kPa	4.7–6.0 kPa
P_aO_2	13.4 kPa	12.0–14.5 kPa

Questions

- What is the cause for this man's coma?
- How would you manage this patient?

ANSWER 89

This man has signs of dehydration, and the high urea with a normal creatinine is consistent with this. He is acidotic. The blood glucose level is not given, but the picture is likely to represent hyperglycaemic ketoacidotic coma. The key clinical features on examination are dehydration shown by skin signs and significant postural hypotension and hyperventilation secondary to a metabolic acidosis, and the triggering problem with the infection in the foot. A persistently high glucose level induced by the response to an infected foot ulcer causes heavy glycosuria, triggering an osmotic diuresis. This leads to hypovolaemia and reduced renal blood flow, causing prerenal uraemia. The extracellular hyperosmolality causes severe cellular dehydration, and loss of water from his brain cells is the cause of his coma. Decreased insulin activity with intracellular glucose deficiency stimulates lipolysis and the production of ketoacids. He has a high anion gap metabolic acidosis due to accumulation of ketoacids (acetoacetate and 3-hydroxybutyrate). The anion gap is calculated from the following equation:

$$[Na^+] + [K^+] - ([Cl^-] + [HCO_3^-])$$

and is normally 10–18 mmol/L; in this case it is 31.5 mmol/L. Ketones cause a characteristically sickly sweet smell on the breath of patients with diabetic ketoacidosis (about 20 per cent of the population cannot smell the ketones). The metabolic acidosis stimulates the respiratory centre, leading to an increase in the rate and depth of respiration (Kussmaul breathing) and producing the reduction in $PaCO_2$ as respiratory compensation for the acidosis. In older diabetic patients there is often evidence of infection (e.g. bronchopneumonia, infected foot ulcer) precipitating these metabolic abnormalities.

The differential diagnosis of coma in diabetics includes non-ketotic hyperglycaemic coma, particularly in elderly diabetics; lactic acidosis, especially in patients on metformin; profound hypoglycaemia; and non-metabolic causes for coma (e.g. cerebrovascular attacks and drug overdose). Salicylate poisoning may cause hyperglycaemia, hyperventilation and coma, but the metabolic picture is usually one of dominant respiratory alkalosis and mild metabolic acidosis.

The aims of management are to correct the massive fluid and electrolyte losses, hyperglycaemia and metabolic acidosis. Rapid fluid replacement with intravenous normal saline and potassium supplements should be started. In patients with cardiac or renal disease, a central venous pressure (CVP) line is needed to control fluid balance. Regular monitoring of plasma potassium is essential, as it may fall very rapidly as glucose enters cells. Insulin therapy is given by intravenous infusion adjusted according to blood glucose levels. A nasogastric tube is used to prevent aspiration of gastric contents, and a bladder catheter is needed to measure urine production. Antibiotics and local wound care should be given to treat this man's foot ulcer. In the longer term it is important that this patient and his wife are educated about his diabetes, and that he has regular access to diabetes services. His smoking and alcohol consumption will also need to be addressed. There may be social issues to be considered in relation to his unemployment.

 KEY POINTS

- Dehydration, tachypnoea and ketosis are the key clinical signs of diabetic ketoacidosis.
- Twenty per cent of the population (and therefore doctors) cannot smell ketones.

CASE 90: COUGH AND BREATHLESSNESS

History

A 69-year-old widower smoked 20 cigarettes a day for over 40 years but then gave them up 9 months ago when his first grandchild was born. He has had a cough with daily sputum production for the last 20 years and has become short of breath over the last 3 years. He coughs up a little white or yellow sputum every morning. He has put on weight recently and now weighs 100 kg. His ankles have become swollen recently, and his exercise tolerance has decreased. He can no longer carry his shopping back from the supermarket 180 m (200 yards) away. He worked as a warehouseman until he was 65 and has become frustrated by his inability to do what he used to do. He is not able to look after his grandchild because he feels too short of breath.

There is no other relevant medical or family history. He lives alone and has a cat and a budgerigar at home.

His general practitioner (GP) gave him a salbutamol metered-dose inhaler, which produced no improvement in his symptoms.

Examination

He is overweight. He appears to be centrally and peripherally cyanosed and has some pitting oedema of his ankles. His jugular venous pressure is raised 3 cm. He has poor chest expansion. There are some early inspiratory crackles at the lung bases.

🔍 INVESTIGATIONS

Respiratory function test results are shown:

	Actual	Predicted
FEV$_1$ (L)	0.55	2.8–3.6
FVC (L)	1.35	3.8–4.6
FER (FEV$_1$/FVC) (%)	41	72–80
PEF (L/min)	90	310–440

FEV$_1$: forced expiratory volume in 1 s; FVC, forced vital capacity; FER, forced expiratory ratio; PEF, peak expiratory flow

---

His chest X-ray is shown in Figure 90.1.

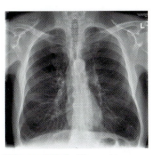

Figure 90.1 Chest X-ray.

Questions

- What is the likely diagnosis?
- What management is appropriate?

ANSWER 90

The most likely diagnosis is chronic obstructive pulmonary disease (COPD). The physical signs and chest X-ray indicate overinflation. The early inspiratory crackles are typical of COPD.

Treatment with bronchodilators should be pursued, looking at the effect of b_2-agonists and anticholinergic agents, judging the effect from the patient's symptoms and exercise tolerance rather than spirometry. Theophylline may sometimes be useful as a third-line therapy but has more side effects.

With this degree of severity, inhaled corticosteroids and long-acting bronchodilators (salmeterol/formoterol or tiotropium) would be appropriate inhaled therapy. Careful attention would need to be given to inhaler technique.

He is cyanosed and has signs of right-sided heart failure (cor pulmonale). Blood gases should be checked to see if he might be a candidate for long-term home oxygen therapy (known to improve survival if the pressure of arterial oxygen (p_aO_2) in the steady-state breathing air remains < 7.2 kPa). Gentle diuresis might help the oedema, although oxygen would be a better approach if he is sufficiently hypoxic. Annual influenza vaccination should be recommended, and *Streptococcus pneumoniae* vaccination should be given. Antibiotics might be kept at home for infective exacerbations.

Exercise tolerance will be reduced by his obesity and by lack of muscle use. A weight-reducing diet should be started. If he has the motivation to continue exercising, then a pulmonary rehabilitation programme has been shown to increase exercise tolerance by around 20 per cent and to improve quality of life. Other more dramatic interventions such as lung reduction surgery or transplantation might be considered in a younger patient. Depression is often associated with the poor exercise tolerance and social isolation, and this should be considered.

COPD is often regarded as a condition for which treatment has little to offer. However, a vigorous approach tailored to the need of the individual patient can provide a worthwhile benefit.

 KEY POINTS

- In COPD β_2-agonists and anticholinergic agents produce similar effects or a greater response from anticholinergics. The combination may be helpful. In contrast, in asthma β_2-agonists produce a greater effect.
- Assessment for home oxygen should be made in a stable state on optimal inhaled therapy.
- Exercise and diet are important elements in the management of COPD.
- Depression is common in chronic conditions such as COPD.

CASE 91: NUMB FEET

History

A 66-year-old man presents with numb feet. In the last few months his feet have felt as though he is wearing thick socks and his feet burn at night. He recently cut his foot whilst walking barefoot in the back garden and didn't feel any pain. He has also been thirstier than usual and has been drinking soft drinks to slake his thirst.

He had an inguinal hernia repaired 2 years ago and he stopped smoking then on the advice of the anaesthetist. Previously he smoked 20 cigarettes per day. He drinks four pints of beer on weekends. His father died of a myocardial infarction at age 58 years.

Examination

His blood pressure is 136/84 mmHg. The respiratory, cardiovascular and abdominal systems are normal. There is a 3 cm ulcerated area with a well-demarcated edge on the dorsum of the right foot. The posterior tibial pulses and dorsalis pedis pulses are palpable. The capillary return time is 2 s. The neurological examination reveals loss of light touch, vibration and pinprick sensation to the ankles. Power in the feet, legs and hands is normal. Ankle jerk is absent bilaterally. Plantar reflexes are down going. There is some loss of pinprick sensation in the hands. The rest of the neurological examination is normal.

INVESTIGATIONS		
		Normal
Haemoglobin	14.3 g/dL	13.7–17.7 g/dL
White cell count	7.4×10^9/L	$3.9–10.6 \times 10^9$/L
Neutrophils	4.6×10^9/L	$1.8–7.7 \times 10^9$/L
Lymphocytes	2.5×10^9/L	$0.6–4.8 \times 10^9$/L
Platelets	372×10^9/L	$150–440 \times 10^9$/L
Sodium	140 mmol/L	135–145 mmol/L
Potassium	4.0 mmol/L	3.5–5.0 mmol/L
Urea	5.1 mmol/L	2.5–6.7 mmol/L
Creatinine	89 μmol/L	70–120 μmol/L
Glucose	12.4 mmol/L	4.0–6.0 mmol/L
HbA$_{1c}$	9.1%	<7%

Question

- What is the likely diagnosis?

ANSWER 91

The glove and stocking distribution of sensory loss with preservation of motor power suggests a peripheral sensory neuropathy. Causes of a peripheral neuropathy are listed in table 91.1. The raised HbA$_{1c}$ suggests diabetes and prolonged hyperglycaemia.

Peripheral neuropathy maybe the first sign of type 2 diabetes mellitus. Initially, sensory loss can be subtle, usually with loss of ankle jerks and vibration in the feet. Sub-clinical neuropathy can be detected using a monofilament. As the neuropathy progresses pinprick sensation is lost and the hands may be involved. In later stages foot deformity can occur. Charcot (neuropathic) joint is caused by repeated joint injury due to the loss of pain sensation. Diabetic neuropathy may lead to unrecognized trauma to the skin which then heals poorly. Diabetic neuropathy and peripheral vascular disease often co-exist and can lead to gangrene.

Further investigations in this patient should include vitamin B12 and folate level, thyroid function, ESR, protein electrophoresis, ANCA and ANA. Genetic tests for an inherited neuropathy or a lead level might be considered if there is a suspicion for these conditions. Alcohol abuse should be apparent from the history but a reduced red blood cell ketolase level can be used to confirm Vitamin B1 (thiamine) deficiency. In diabetic neuropathy, nerve conduction studies are rarely needed, but may be helpful to exclude an entrapment neuropathy such as carpel tunnel syndrome. Co-existing peripheral vascular disease is common in diabetes and measurement of the ankle:brachial blood pressure ratio should be performed if there are absent lower limb pulses. A value less than 0.97 it suggests arterial disease. The development of one diabetic complication should prompt the search for other complications: diabetic retinopathy; nephropathy; coronary and carotid vascular disease.

Table 91.1 Causes of peripheral neuropathy

- Diabetes mellitus
- Carcinoma
- Critical illness
- Drugs (including amiodarone, cisplatin, isoniazid, metronidazole, nitrofurantion, vincristine)
- Toxins (alcohol, arsenic, lead, thallium)
- Genetic (Charcot–Marie–Tooth disease, Fabry's disease, Friedrich's ataxia)
- Vitamin deficiencies (vitamin B1-thiamine, vitamin B3-niacin, vitamin B6-pyrodoxine, vitamin B12-cyanocobalamin)
- Uraemia
- Chronic liver disease
- HIV
- Lymphoma
- Multiple myeloma
- Benign monoclonal gammopathy
- Primary systemic amyloidosis

Treatment of type 2 diabetes mellitus includes dietary advice, oral hypoglycaemics and possibly insulin. The goal is for a HbA$_{1c}$ less than 7.5%. Blood glucose control can slow further progression of diabetic neuropathy. Prevention of diabetic foot ulcers is essential and should include use of comfortable shoes, avoiding bare feet, regular chiropody and aggressive treatment of nail infections. Diabetic neuropathy that is painful may benefit from amitryptiline, gabapentin or topical capsaicin cream. Antibiotics and specialist dressings may be required if foot ulcers develop. A total contact cast to offload pressure on the foot is particularly helpful for neuropathic ulcers. Osteomyelitis is common in deep ulcers. MRI is the investigation of choice. Regular follow-up of patients with type 2 diabetes to prevent foot disease should include neurological and vascular examination of both feet and testing for peripheral neuropathy with a monofilament.

KEY POINTS

- Peripheral neuropathy maybe the first presentation of type 2 diabetes mellitus.
- Diabetic feet are particularly vulnerable because of sensory loss, arterial insufficiency and high sugars.

CASE 92: A HEALTHY MAN?

History

A 50-year-old man has a health screen as part of an application for life insurance. He has no symptoms. He smokes 15 cigarettes per day and drinks 10 units of alcohol per week. In his family history his father died of a myocardial infarction at age 56 years.

Examination

He weighs 84 kg and is 1.6 m (5 ft, 8 in.) tall. His blood pressure is 164/98 mmHg. Examination is otherwise normal.

🔍 INVESTIGATIONS

		Normal
Haemoglobin	15.2 g/dL	13.3–17.7 g/dL
White cell count	10.0×10^9/L	$3.9–10.6 \times 10^9$/L
Platelets	287×10^9/L	$150–440 \times 10^9$/L
Sodium	139 mmol/L	135–145 mmol/L
Potassium	3.9 mmol/L	3.5–5.0 mmol/L
Urea	4.3 mmol/L	2.5–6.7 mmol/L
Creatinine	88 µmol/L	70–120 µmol/L
Cholesterol	5.0 mmol/L	<5.5 mmol/L
Triglyceride	1.30 mmol/L	0.55–1.90 mmol/L
Very low-density lipoprotein (VLDL)	0.44 mmol/L	0.12–0.65 mmol/L
Low-density lipoprotein (LDL)	3.1 mmol/L	1.6–4.4 mmol/L
High-density lipoprotein (HDL)	1.9 mmol/L	0.9–1.9 mmol/L

His electrocardiogram (ECG) is shown in Figure 92.1.

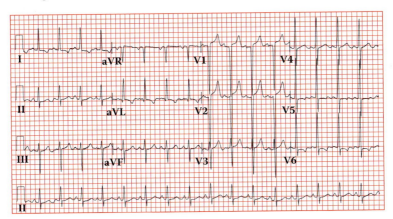

Figure 92.1 Electrocardiogram.

Question

- What is the appropriate management?

ANSWER 92

The ECG shows left ventricular hypertrophy (R-wave in V5 and S-wave in V1 >35 mm). Although only a single reading is given, the hypertrophy makes it likely that the blood pressure represents sustained hypertension rather than a 'white coat' effect. Blood pressure readings should be repeated or 24 h blood pressure monitoring should be performed before treatment is started. The diagnosis of hypertension based upon ambulatory blood pressure monitoring is a 24 h average above 130/85; daytime average above 140/90 and nighttime average above 125/75.

The risks of vascular disease are related to the presence of other risk factors. The body mass index is 28, showing that he is overweight. He is a smoker with a positive family history of cardiovascular disease. Tables such as the Sheffield table can be used to obtain a calculation of the risks of cardiovascular disease.

The other question is whether a search for the cause of the hypertension is indicated. Around 85 per cent of cases are idiopathic. Most of the secondary cases are related to renal disease, and the renal function is normal here. A number of endocrine causes (Cushing's syndrome, Conn's syndrome) are associated with hypokalaemia. If the blood pressure is difficult to control, secondary causes such as renal artery stenosis should be considered and investigated by renal ultrasound or a technique to visualize the renal arteries, such as magnetic resonance angiography or digital subtraction angiography. Obstructive sleep apnea can also cause resistant hypertension.

The cholesterol is at a level that would warrant treatment if there was evidence of vascular disease. The hypertension itself should be controlled according to current guidelines, which would recommend starting with an angiotensin-converting enzyme (ACE) inhibitor in a patient younger than 55 years.

 KEY POINTS

- A single elevated blood pressure needs to be remeasured over several weeks.
- All relevant risk factors should be considered in assessing cardiovascular risk and planning treatment.
- Most cases of hypertension do not have an identifiable underlying cause.

CASE 93: TIREDNESS

History

A 79-year-old man is brought to his general practitioner by his daughter, who says that he is getting very tired and has lost interest in life. She says that a general malaise has been present for 5–6 weeks. She thinks that he might have lost a few kilograms in weight over this time, but he does not weigh himself regularly. He says that he has felt limited on exertion by tiredness for a year or so, and on a few occasions when he tried to do more, he had a feeling of tightness across his chest. There is no other medical history of note. He smokes 20 cigarettes a day and drinks a pint or two of Guinness each Saturday and Sunday. He is not on any medication and just takes paracetamol occasionally. On systems review, he says that he has lost his appetite over the last month. His sleep has been disturbed by occasional nocturia, and on two or three occasions in the last few weeks, he has been disturbed by sweating at night.

There is no relevant family history. He is a retired shopkeeper who normally keeps reasonably fit walking his dog.

Examination

His pulse is 70/min; blood pressure is 110/66 mmHg. There is no clubbing, but tar staining is present on the fingers and nails of the right hand. The jugular venous pressure is not raised. The apex beat is displaced 2 cm from the midclavicular line. On auscultation of the heart there is a grade 3/6 ejection systolic murmur radiating to the carotids and a soft early diastolic murmur audible at the lower left sternal edge. There are no abnormalities to find in the abdomen or nervous system. The urine looked clear, but routine stick testing showed a trace of blood, and on urine microscopy there were some red cells. A chest X-ray was reported as showing a slightly large heart.

🔍 INVESTIGATIONS

		Normal
Haemoglobin	10.7 g/dL	13.3–17.7 g/dL
Mean corpuscular volume (MCV)	88 fL	80–99 fL
White cell count	12.2×10^9/L	$3.9–10.6 \times 10^9$/L
Neutrophils	10.5×10^9/L	$1.8–7.7 \times 10^9$/L
Lymphocytes	1.5×10^9/L	$0.6–4.8 \times 10^9$/L
Platelets	287×10^9/L	$150–440 \times 10^9$/L
Erythrocyte sedimentation rate (ESR)	68 mm in 1 h	<20 mm in 1 h

The electrocardiogram (ECG) is shown in Figure 93.1.

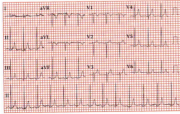

Figure 93.1 Electrocardiogram.

Questions

- What is the most likely diagnosis?
- What investigations are indicated?

ANSWER 93

This 79-year-old man has the clinical features of aortic stenosis and regurgitation. The murmurs are of mixed aortic valve disease and the ECG shows left ventricular hypertrophy (sum of negative deflection in V1 and positive deflection in V5 or V2 and V6 greater than 35 mm), suggesting that there has been significant pressure overload from aortic stenosis. The findings of mixed aortic valve disease, microscopic haematuria, malaise and fever (probable with the history of night sweats) make it likely that the diagnosis is infective endocarditis. This would also fit with the haematological picture showing normocytic anaemia, raised neutrophil count and a high ESR. In the elderly, infective endocarditis may be an insidious illness and should be considered in any patient who has murmurs and fever or any other change in the cardiac signs or symptoms. The other classical findings of splenomegaly, splinter haemorrhages, clubbing, Osler's nodes, Janeway lesions and Roth's spots are usually absent. Precipitating events such as dental treatment or other sources of bacteraemia may not be evident in the history.

It is difficult to tie all the features into any other single diagnosis. The signs are of aortic valve disease. When there is a fever or other evidence of infection in the presence of valve disease, infective endocarditis must always be considered, although in practice other unrelated infections are more common. Other infections, such as tuberculosis or abscess, are possible, or there could be an underlying lymphoma or other malignancy.

The most important investigations would be the following:

- blood cultures performed before any antibiotics are given. In this case three blood cultures grew *Streptococcus viridans.*
- echocardiogram, which showed a thickened bicuspid aortic valve, a common congenital abnormality predisposing to significant functional valve disturbance in middle and old age. Vegetations can be detected on a transthoracic echocardiogram if they are prominent; at transoesophageal echocardiogram is more sensitive in detecting vegetations on the valves but more demanding for the patient and the operator.

Treatment with intravenous benzylpenicillin and gentamicin for 2 weeks, followed by oral amoxicillin resulted in resolution of the fever with no haemodynamic deterioration or change in the murmurs of mixed aortic valve disease. A microbiologist should be consulted about appropriate antibiotics and duration.

After treatment of the endocarditis, the symptoms of pain and tiredness on exertion would need to be considered to see if valve surgery was indicated. Prior to this it would be routine to look at the coronary arteries by angiography to see if simultaneous coronary artery surgery was needed in a patient of this age.

 KEY POINTS

- Symptoms on exertion in aortic valve disease are a sign that valve surgery needs to be considered.
- In infective endocarditis, it is unusual to have many of the classical physical signs. In the elderly, it may present with non-specific malaise.

CASE 94: ABDOMINAL PAIN

History

A 70-year-old woman is admitted to hospital with acute onset of abdominal pain. The abdominal pain started quite suddenly 24 h before admission and has continued since then. It is a constant central abdominal pain. She has vomited altered food on one occasion.

She has a history of occasional angina on exertion for 5 years. She has a glyceryl trinitrate spray, but she has not needed this in the last 3 months. A year ago she was found to be in atrial fibrillation at 120/min, and she was started on digoxin, which she still takes. The only other medical history of note is that she had a hysterectomy for menorrhagia 30 years ago, and she has hypertension controlled on a small dose of a thiazide diuretic for the last 3 years. She does not take any other medication apart from low-dose aspirin. She does not smoke and does not drink alcohol. She retired from work as a cleaner 8 years ago.

Examination

She was in atrial fibrillation at a rate of 92/min with a blood pressure of 114/76 mmHg. Respiratory examination was normal. She was tender with some guarding in the centre of the abdomen. No masses were palpable in the abdomen, and there were just occasional bowel sounds to hear on auscultation. Over the next 2 h the blood pressure fell to 84/60 mmHg. She was admitted to the intensive care unit (ICU) and monitored while initial investigations were performed. The abdominal X-ray showed no gas under the diaphragm and no dilated loops of bowel or fluid levels. While under observation, the urine output fell off. Re-examination showed that bowel sounds were absent. Her hands and feet remained warm. Measurements of cardiac output in the ICU showed that it remained high.

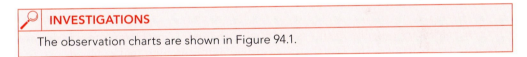

INVESTIGATIONS

The observation charts are shown in Figure 94.1.

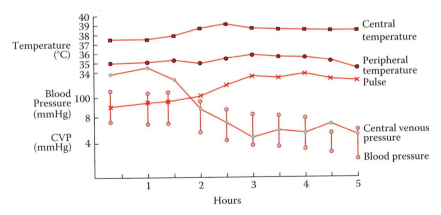

Figure 94.1 Chart from intensive care unit.

Questions

- What is the likely cause of the abdominal pain?
- What further developments do the charts suggest?

ANSWER 94

One diagnosis of the abdominal pain that would explain her condition and fit with her predisposing situation is ischaemic bowel caused by an embolus from the heart. The patient is likely to become very ill without markedly abnormal physical signs. Atrial fibrillation increases the likelihood of such an event. She has been on aspirin, which will reduce slightly the risk of embolic events, but is not on anticoagulants, which would have decreased the risk further. In the presence of pre-existing cardiovascular problems, shown by the hypertension and angina, anticoagulation would normally be started if there are no contraindications. The risk of cerebrovascular accidents caused by emboli from the heart has been shown to be reduced. In lone atrial fibrillation with no underlying cardiac disease, the risks of emboli and the benefits of anticoagulation are less. There are alternative diagnoses, such as perforation or pancreatitis, and it is not possible to be sure of the cause of the abdominal problem from the information given here.

The chart of the observations (Figure 94.1) covers 10 h. After the first hour or two the central venous pressure drops, the blood pressure falls, and the pulse rate rises in association with the fall in urine output.

These findings show that she is developing shock with inadequate perfusion of vital organs.

> **! Possible causes for shock**
>
> | Types of shock | Example |
> | --- | --- |
> | Hypovolaemic shock | Blood loss |
> | Cardiogenic shock | Myocardial infarction |
> | Extracardiac obstructive shock | Pulmonary embolism |
> | Vasodilatory (distributive) shock | Sepsis |

All these causes are possible in this woman with abdominal problems and a history of ischaemic heart disease. The fact that the cardiac output is high makes blood loss and cardiogenic shock unlikely. The most likely cause is septic shock, for which peripheral vasodilation would lead to a high cardiac output but a falling blood pressure and rising pulse rate. Vasoconstriction and reduced blood flow occur in certain organs, such as the kidneys, leading to the term *distributive shock* with maintained overall cardiac output but inappropriate distribution of blood flow. The rise in central temperature and the lack of a marked fall in peripheral temperature would fit with this cause of the shock.

The patient was stabilized with fluid replacement and antibiotics before going to theatre, where the diagnosis of ischaemic bowel from an embolus was confirmed. Arteriography can confirm the diagnosis, but confirmation is often at laparotomy, which is usually required to remove the necrotic bowel.

> **KEY POINTS**
>
> - Aspirin and anticoagulation should be considered in patients with atrial fibrillation.
> - Septic shock may be present with warm peripheries through vasodilation.
> - A drop in the central venous pressure may be the first sign of developing shock.

CASE 95: CLUMSINESS

History

A 66-year-old woman notices that she is having trouble performing some everyday tasks, such as doing up buttons on her blouse and chopping vegetables for cooking. She complains that her muscles feel stiff, and it is taking her longer than it did to walk to the local shops. She is anxious about these problems since she lives alone and has to do everything for herself. She has noticed a little shakiness, which she ascribes to anxiety. Her daughter has told her that it is becoming increasingly difficult to read the small writing in the letters she sends. She is a retired journalist and has no significant past medical history. There is no disturbance of her bowels or micturition. Her appetite has been good and her weight steady. She complains that she has been sleeping poorly and is consequently rather tired. She does not smoke tobacco and drinks only occasionally. She has hypertension and takes 50 mg atenolol daily.

Examination

Her pulse is 60/min and regular; blood pressure is 134/84 mmHg. There are no abnormalities in the cardiovascular or respiratory systems. On neurological examination there is no muscle wasting. She has generally increased muscle tone throughout the range of movement, equal in flexors and extensors. There is a slight tremor affecting mainly her right hand, which is suppressed when she tries to do something. She has problems with fine tasks such as doing up buttons. Power, reflexes, coordination and sensation are all normal. When asked to walk she is a little slow to get started and has difficulty stopping and turning.

Questions
- What is the diagnosis?
- How would you investigate and manage this patient?

ANSWER 95

There is evidence in the history and examination of tremor, rigidity and bradykinesia. Her writing shows micrographia secondary to the rigidity and slowness of movement. Her hypertension is well controlled on the beta-blocker. Beta-blockers can cause tiredness and slowness but not to the extent seen in this woman. This woman has Parkinson's disease presenting with the classic triad of tremor, rigidity and hypokinesia. Tremor is usually an early symptom and may be unilateral. The combination of tremor with rigidity leads to the cogwheel form of rigidity. The patient often goes on to have a blank mask-like facies. There is difficulty starting to walk (freezing), and the patient uses small steps and has difficulty stopping (festination). There is generally normal intellectual function, but there is often depression. Sleep is often disturbed, contributing to daytime tiredness. The characteristic pathological abnormality is degeneration of dopamine-secreting neurones in the nigrostriatal pathway of the basal ganglia.

Parkinsonian features (parkinsonism) may occur in a variety of diseases:

- Parkinson's disease
- postencephalitic parkinsonism
- neuroleptic drug-induced Parkinson's disease
- parkinsonism in association with Alzheimer's/multi-infarct dementia.

! Classification of tremor

- *Rest tremor*: the tremor is worse at rest and is typical of parkinsonism.
- *Postural tremor*: this is characteristic of benign essential tremor, physiological tremor and exaggerated physiological tremor caused by anxiety, alcohol and thyrotoxicosis. Benign essential tremor is not present at rest, but appears on holding the arms outstretched, but is not worse on movement (finger–nose testing). Tests of coordination are normal, and walking is unaffected. There is usually a family history of tremor, and the tremor is helped by alcohol and beta-blockers.
- *Intention tremor*: the tremor is worse on movement and is most obvious in finger–nose testing. It is usually caused by brainstem or cerebellar disease caused by such diseases as multiple sclerosis, localized tumours or spinocerebellar degeneration.

A variety of drugs are available to treat this woman's Parkinson's disease. Selegiline, an inhibitor of monoamine oxidase B, may delay the need to start levodopa and may slow the rate of progression of the disease but has significant side effects. Levodopa is usually used in combination with a selective dopa decarboxylase inhibitor, which does not cross the blood–brain barrier and reduces peripheral adverse effects. The commonest side effects are nausea, vomiting, dizziness, postural hypotension and neuropsychiatric problems. After many years of treatment the effects tend to diminish, and the patient may develop rapid oscillations in control—the 'on–off' effect. When these develop, a sustained-release formulation of levodopa or a dopamine agonist (e.g. bromocriptine) may produce improvement. Because of the loss of effect with time, treatment should not be started too early. This requires careful discussion with the individual patient. She should be assessed by a physiotherapist and occupational therapist and provided with advice and aids. With time her house may need to be altered to aid her mobility.

KEY POINTS

- Parkinson's disease is characterized by tremor, rigidity and hypokinesia.
- Patient management is long term and multidisciplinary.
- Benefits of levodopa treatment in Parkinson's disease may lessen with time.

CASE 96: SHORTNESS OF BREATH

History

A 35-year-old woman presents with a 6-month history of increasing shortness of breath. This has progressed so that she is now short of breath on walking up one flight of stairs and walks more slowly on the flat than other people her age. In addition she has developed a dry cough over the last 3 months.

In her previous medical history, she had mild asthma as a child. She thinks that her father died of a chest problem in his 40s. She takes occasional paracetamol and has taken 'slimming pills' in the past.

She is a lifetime non-smoker and drinks less than 10 units of alcohol per week. She has worked in the printing trade since she left school. She has two children, aged 8 and 10 years, and they have a cat and a rabbit at home.

Examination

There is no clubbing, anaemia or cyanosis. Examination of the cardiovascular system is normal. In the respiratory system, expansion of the lungs seems to be reduced but symmetrical. The percussion note is normal, as is tactile vocal fremitus. On auscultation there are some fine late inspiratory crackles at both lung bases.

🔍 INVESTIGATIONS

Respiratory function tests revealed the following:

	Actual	Predicted
FEV$_1$ (L)	3.0	3.6–4.2
FVC (L)	3.6	4.5–5.3
FER (FEV$_1$/FVC) (%)	83	75–80
PEF (L/min)	470	450–550

FEV$_1$: forced expiratory volume in 1 s; FVC, forced vital capacity; FER, forced expiratory ratio; PEF, peak expiratory flow.

Her chest X-ray is shown in Figure 96.1 and a high-resolution computed tomography (CT) scan in Figure 96.2.

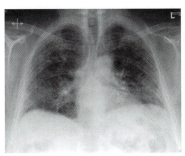

Figure 96.1 Chest X-ray.

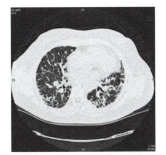

Figure 96.2 High-resolution computed tomography scan.

Questions

- What is the likely diagnosis?
- What further investigations and treatment are indicated?

ANSWER 96

The history shows a progressive condition over at least 6 months. It is often difficult to be sure of the exact length of history when a symptom such as breathlessness has an insidious onset. A few possibilities are raised by the details of the history. There is a history of asthma, but the absence of wheezing or obstruction on the respiratory function tests rule that out as the cause of the current problem. An occupational history is always important in lung disease but probably not here. Occupational asthma can be associated with isocyanates used in the printing trade but this would cause an obstructive problem rather than the restrictive problem shown here. The findings on examination fit with a restrictive problem with limited expansion and crackles caused by reopening of airways closing during expiration because of stiff lungs and low lung volumes.

The respiratory function tests show a mild restrictive ventilatory defect with reduced FEV_1 and FVC but a slightly high ratio, suggesting stiff lungs or chest wall. Further tests such as transfer factor would be expected to be reduced in the presence of pulmonary fibrosis.

The chest X-ray shows small lung fields and nodular and reticular shadowing most marked in mid- and lower zones. The high-resolution CT scan shows widespread fibrotic change with subpleural cyst formation. These changes are compatible with diffuse pulmonary fibrosis (fibrosing alveolitis). In talking about fibrosis of the lungs, it is important to differentiate diffuse fine pulmonary fibrosis, as in this case, and localized pulmonary fibrosis as a result of scarring after an acute inflammatory condition, such as pneumonia. The distribution and the pattern of the changes on the CT scan are important in determining the diagnosis and the likelihood of response to treatment in pulmonary fibrosis. Diffuse pulmonary fibrosis can be associated with conditions such as rheumatoid arthritis and can be induced by inhaled dusts or ingested drugs. None of these seem likely here, making this likely to be idiopathic pulmonary fibrosis (IPF). There is a rare familial form, so the father's illness might be relevant. The most common type of IPF is usual interstitial pneumonia (UIP) with a subpleural distribution on the CT scan as shown here. In association with connective tissue disease, there may be a more widespread patchy pattern of non-specific interstitial pneumonitis (NSIP). The appearance of 'ground-glass' shadowing on the high-resolution CT is associated with active cellular alveolitis and the greater likelihood of response to treatment. NSIP also has a better response rate than UIP.

Further investigations consist of a search for a cause or associated conditions and a decision whether a lung biopsy is warranted. Bronchoscopic biopsies are too small to be representative or useful in this situation, and a video-assisted thoracoscopic biopsy would be the usual procedure. It would usually be appropriate to obtain histology of the lung in someone of this age.

Treatment consists of low- to moderate-dose corticosteroids with or without an immunosuppressant such as azathioprine continued for several months to look for an effect, but the results are poor in UIP, and it is important not to cause more harm than benefit from treatment with prolonged steroids and immunosuppressants. There is some evidence that antioxidants such as acetylcysteine improve the outlook, and these may be combined with the steroids and azathioprine and new agents are under investigation. In a patient of this age, lung transplantation might be a consideration as the disease progresses. Progression rates are variable, and an acute aggressive form with death in 6 months can occur. More common in UIP is steady progression over a few years.

KEY POINTS

- Diffuse pulmonary fibrosis has a range of causes relevant to management.
- Ineffective treatment may produce serious side effects without significant benefit.

CASE 97: ROUTINE FOLLOW-UP

History

Four months ago a 47-year-old publican was admitted to hospital with acute chest pain. A subendocardial inferior myocardial infarction was diagnosed, and he was treated with thrombolytics and aspirin. After discharge he complained of angina, and a coronary angiography was performed. This showed severe triple-vessel disease not suitable for stenting, and coronary artery bypass grafting was performed. He is attending a cardiac rehabilitation clinic, and he has had no further angina since his surgery. He has a strong family history of ischaemic heart disease, with his father and two paternal uncles having died of myocardial infarctions in their 50s; his 50-year-old brother has angina. He is married with two children. He smokes 25 cigarettes per day and drinks at least 40 units of alcohol per week. He is taking atenolol and aspirin.

Examination

He is slightly overweight (85 kg; body mass index = 28 kg/m²). He has tar-stained nails. He has bilateral corneal arcus, xanthelasmata around his eyes and xanthomata on his Achilles tendons. He has a well-healed midline sternotomy scar. His pulse is 64/min and regular; blood pressure is 150/84 mmHg. He has no palpable pedal pulses. His respiratory, gastrointestinal and neurological systems are normal.

INVESTIGATIONS		
		Normal
Haemoglobin	16.2 g/dL	13.3–17.7 g/dL
White cell count	10.0 × 10⁹/L	3.9–10.6 × 10⁹/L
Platelets	336 × 10⁹/L	150–440 × 10⁹/L
Sodium	135 mmol/L	135–145 mmol/L
Potassium	3.9 mmol/L	3.5–5.0 mmol/L
Urea	3.4 mmol/L	2.5–6.7 mmol/L
Creatinine	82 µmol/L	70–120 µmol/L
Bilirubin	16 mmol/L	3–17 mmol/L
Alanine transaminase	33 IU/L	5–35 IU/L
Alkaline phosphatase	72 IU/L	30–300 IU/L
Gamma-glutamyl transpeptidase	68 IU/L	11–51 IU/L
Cholesterol	12.2 mmol/L	<5.5 mmol/L
Triglyceride	2.30 mmol/L	0.55–1.90 mmol/L
Very low-density lipoprotein (VLDL)	0.34 mmol/L	0.13–0.65 mmol/L
Low-density lipoprotein (LDL)	8.5 mmol/L	1.6–4.4 mmol/L
High-density lipoprotein (HDL)	0.6 mmol/L	0.9–1.9 mmol/L

Urinalysis: no abnormality detected

Questions

- What is the metabolic abnormality present?
- What advice would you give this man?

ANSWER 97

The obvious abnormality in the investigation is a very high serum cholesterol with high LDL and low HDL levels. He has many clinical features to go with the high cholesterol and premature vascular disease. This man has familial hypercholesterolaemia. He has presented with premature coronary artery disease. His absent pedal pulses suggest peripheral vascular disease. Familial hypercholesterolaemia is an autosomal dominant condition. The homozygous condition is rare, and affected individuals usually die before the age of 20 years due to premature atherosclerosis. The heterozygous form affects about 1 in 400 individuals in the United Kingdom, and 50 per cent of males will develop ischaemic heart disease before the age of 50 years. Corneal arcus, xanthelasmata and xanthomata on Achilles tendons and the extensor tendons on the dorsum of the hands develop in early adult life. The metabolic defect is a result of a reduced number of high-affinity cell-surface LDL receptors. This leads to increased LDL levels. Increased uptake of LDL by macrophage scavenger receptors leads to increased oxidized LDL, which is particularly atherogenic. Triglyceride and VLDL levels are normal or mildly elevated. HDL levels are low. The other major causes of hypercholesterolaemia are familial combined hyperlipidaemia and polygenic hypercholesterolaemia. Familial combined hyperlipidaemia differs from familial hypercholesterolaemia in patients having raised triglycerides. Patients with polygenic hypercholesterolaemia have a similar lipid profile to familial hypercholesterolaemia but they do not develop xanthomata. Hypercholesterolaemia may commonly occur in hypothyroidism, diabetes mellitus, nephrotic syndrome and hepatic cholestasis.

This patient is at extremely high risk for further vascular events, especially occlusion of his coronary artery bypass grafts. His risk depends on the combination of his risk factors, and all of these need attention. He should be advised to stop smoking, reduce his alcohol intake (which is also affecting his liver, as judged from the raised gamma-glutamyl transpeptidase), take more exercise, and eat a strict low-cholesterol diet. Diet alone will not control this level of cholesterol. He should have pharmacological treatment with a statin but may need combined treatment for this level of hyperlipidaemia. His children should have their lipid profile measured so that they can be treated to prevent premature coronary artery disease. There is clear evidence from clinical trials that primary prevention of coronary artery disease can be achieved by lowering serum cholesterol. The West of Scotland Coronary Prevention Study (WOSCOPS) showed cholesterol lowering with pravastatin reduced both the number of coronary events and coronary mortality in middle-aged men with a serum LDL level greater than 4 mmol/L. In patients who have evidence of cardiovascular disease, secondary prevention is even more important, aiming for a cholesterol level as low as possible. Statins are well tolerated, although myositis is a rare but serious complication.

 KEY POINTS

- The commonest causes for hypercholesterolaemia are polygenic hypercholesterolaemia, familial hypercholesterolaemia and familial combined hyperlipidaemia.
- Effective drugs are now available to treat hypercholesterolaemia and should be used aggressively to reduce coronary artery disease.
- In secondary prevention the aim is the lowest possible cholesterol level.

CASE 98: CHANGE IN CHARACTER

History

A 66-year-old man has been persuaded by his wife to go to his general practitioner (GP). She is worried that he has changed. Over the last 4 weeks he has become lethargic and rather vague. He has a 12-year history of chronic cough and sputum production, but she thinks that these symptoms may have increased a little over the last 8 weeks. He has smoked 20 cigarettes daily for the last 50 years, and he drinks around 14 units of alcohol per week. Two years ago he became depressed and was treated with an antidepressant for 6 months with good effect. She cannot remember the name of the medication. He had worked all his life as a postman until retirement 6 years ago.

Examination

He is a little vague in his answers to questions. There are no abnormalities in the cardio-vascular, respiratory or abdominal systems. There is no lymphadenopathy. On neurological examination he seems to have mild generalized muscle weakness. Reflexes, tone and sensation are all normal. His peak flow and spirometry measures are within normal limits.

INVESTIGATIONS		
		Normal
Haemoglobin	14.8 g/dL	13.0–17.0 g/dL
Mean corpuscular volume (MCV)	86 fL	80–99 fL
White cell count	6.9 × 10⁹/L	4.0–11.0 × 10⁹/L
Platelets	297 × 10⁹/L	150–400 × 10⁹/L
Sodium	119 mmol/L	135–150 mmol/L
Potassium	3.5 mmol/L	3.4–5.0 mmol/L
Urea	3.1 mmol/L	2.5–7.5 mmol/L
Creatinine	63 µmol/L	70–120 µmol/L

His chest X-ray is shown in Figure 98.1.

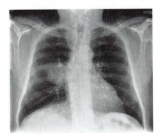

Figure 98.1 Chest X-ray.

Questions
- How do you interpret these findings?
- What would be the appropriate management?

ANSWER 98

The blood results show hyponatraemia, and the chest X-ray shows a mass overlying the right hilum. This degree of hyponatraemia might be expected to cause some cerebral changes. A lower level might be associated with seizures. Above 120–125 mmol/L, the effects are likely to be non-specific tiredness.

Possible causes for the hyponatraemia in this man are

- inappropriate arginine vasopressin (AVP, antidiuretic hormone) secretion in association with the respiratory disorders of undifferentiated small-cell carcinoma of the lung or, occasionally, with pneumonia or tuberculosis; or
- Addison's disease (adrenocortical failure), which would be expected to produce a high potassium level and postural hypotension. Addison's disease might be linked with respiratory problems through adrenal involvement by metastases or tuberculosis.

Other causes, such as diuretic treatment; inappropriate AVP from drug therapy (e.g. carbamazepine, phenothiazines, amitriptyline); cerebrovascular events; salt-losing nephropathies; or overhydration from intravenous fluids or overdrinking are not likely from the story given here. He has been treated with antidepressants, but not for the last 18 months. In view of the chest X-ray, the most likely diagnosis is inappropriate AVP secretion with a small-cell undifferentiated carcinoma of the lung. This can be confirmed by measurement of serum and urine osmolarities to show serum dilution while the urine is concentrated. Levels of AVP can be measured.

In this case, the osmolarities confirmed the syndrome of inappropriate antidiuretic hormone secretion (SIADH); bronchial biopsies at fibre-optic bronchoscopy showed a small-cell undifferentiated carcinoma. Extension to the carina and computed tomography (CT) appearances showed it was not resectable. Fluid restriction to 750 mL daily produced an increase in serum sodium to128 mmol/L with improvement in the confusion and weakness. If this fails to produce adequate results, demeclocycline can be used. This derivative of tetracycline antibiotics interferes with the action of ADH in the renal tubules. Vasopressin antagonists such as tolvaptan are also effective at raising serum sodium, but they are expensive and can cause over-rapid correction.

Chemotherapy was started for the lung tumour. Such treatment often produces a response in terms of shrinkage of the tumour, improved quality of life and increased survival. It may also help the ectopic hormone secretion. Unfortunately, cure is still infrequent. Small-cell undifferentiated carcinomas of the lung are fast-growing tumours, usually unresectable at presentation.

 KEY POINTS

- Change of character may have a metabolic explanation.
- The commonest cause of hyponatraemia is diuretic therapy.
- Measurement of serum and urine osmolarities can help to determine the cause of hyponatraemia.

CASE 99: SHORTNESS OF BREATH

History

A 20-year-old woman has complained of intermittent shortness of breath with wheezing and cough for 3 years. She had eczema and rhinitis up to 8 years of age. A diagnosis of asthma was made but control of her symptoms has been difficult and she is now being treated with salbutamol, salmeterol, high dose inhaled corticosteroids and montelukast. The breathlessness is intermittent. When the breathlessness comes on she feels unable to take air into her lungs, and is often unable to speak and finds that multiple doses of salbutamol provide little relief. She presents to the accident and emergency department with an acute exacerbation of her breathlessness.

Examination

She is unable to speak in more than a whisper. Her respiratory rate is 26/min. Pulse rate is 92/min and blood pressure 128/84 mmHg. Her temperature is 36.8°C and oxygen saturation is 98% on air. The heart sounds are normal. There is a generalized inspiratory and expiratory wheeze heard all over the chest but no other abnormalities. She finds it difficult to perform a peak flow recording but manages 60 L/min.

🔍 INVESTIGATIONS

After recovery from this acute episode she is sent for respiratory function tests which show:

	Actual	Postbronchodilator	Predicted
FEV_1 (L)	3.5	3.7	3.5–4.3
FVC (L)	4.6	4.8	4.6–5.4
FER (FEV_1/FVC) (%)	76	77	72–80
PEF (L/min)	440	480	440–540

FEV_1: forced expiratory volume in 1 s; FVC, forced vital capacity; FER, forced expiratory ratio; PEF, peak expiratory flow.

Question

• What is the most likely diagnosis?

ANSWER 99

This woman has intermittent breathlessness with wheezing. Much the commonest cause of these symptoms would be asthma but there are a number of features which make this less likely in this patient.

Loss of voice is a prominent symptom. The history suggests little response to beta agonist treatment, and the lung function tests after recovery from the episode do not show airflow obstruction or a significant response to bronchodilators. The airway narrowing in asthma may be intermittent showing no obstruction between attacks, in which case it may be necessary to look for increased bronchial responsiveness to a challenge such as exercise or inhaled methacholine.

During the acute episode in association with severe symptoms the oxygen saturation is, surprisingly, normal. Inability to speak in complete sentences is a characteristic of severe asthma but the loss of voice here suggests that there may be a problem at vocal cord level and this would fit with the marked inspiratory and expiratory wheezing and the feeling of being unable to take air into her lungs although asthmatics may complain of similar problems.

These features suggest that the diagnosis of vocal cord dysfunction is more likely than asthma in this woman. In this condition there is paradoxical motion of the vocal cords so that they adduct on inspiration to produce inspiratory airflow obstruction at the level of the larynx. Episodes of breathlessness tend to be intermittent, unresponsive to conventional asthma treatment and associated with stridor.

The most important diagnostic tests are direct viewing of the cords by an ear nose and throat surgeon and a flow volume loop. Inspection of the cords will show paradoxical motion and adduction of the anterior cords with a posterior 'glottis chink' allowing limited airflow. A flow volume loop will show a relatively normal expiratory phase but loss of flow or low flow in the latter part of the inspiratory loop as the vocal cords adduct and produce obstruction (Figure 99.1). In asthma, obstruction would be evident in both expiratory and inspiratory limbs of the flow volume loop.

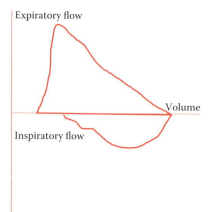

Figure 99.1 Flow–volume loop showing cutoff of inspiratory flow in vocal cord dysfunction.

It is important to recognise this condition so that inappropriate treatment for asthma can be stopped and appropriate treatment can be started. Vocal cord dysfunction is present in around 10% of patients with refractory asthma. It is more common in the presence of psychiatric problems such as depression and anxiety and may be associated with gastro-oesophageal reflux which should be treated. The mainstays of treatment are speech therapy, relaxation and breathing techniques.

 KEY POINTS

- When asthma is difficult to control other diagnoses such as vocal cord dysfunction or large airway obstruction should be considered.
- Flow volume loops may be useful in differentiating causes of airflow obstruction.

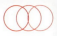

CASE 100: KIDNEY FAILURE

History

A 48-year-old woman is seen by her GP complaining of tiredness for several months. She also has suffered from headaches over the past 6 weeks for which she has been taking regular ibuprofen. She has no significant past medical history. She has two children aged 16 and 13. Her pregnancies were uncomplicated. She has complained of painful periods over many years for which she has taken a variety of non-steroidal inflammatory drugs and over-the-counter herbal remedies.

Examination

She looks pale. Her pulse is 84/min regular, blood pressure 178/102 mmHg, jugular venous pressure not raised, heart sounds normal. Her respiratory and abdominal examinations are normal. Neurological examination is normal. Funduscopy shows arteriovenous nipping and silver-wiring of the retinal vessels.

🔍 INVESTIGATIONS

		Normal
Haemoglobin	12.0 g/dL	11.7–15.7 g/dL
White cell count	10.8 × 10⁹/L	3.5–11.0 × 10⁹/L
Platelets	154 × 10⁹/L	150–440 × 10⁹/L
Sodium	137 mmol/L	135–145 mmol/L
Potassium	4.8 mmol/L	3.5–5.0 mmol/L
Urea	12.1 mmol/L	2.5–6.7 mmol/L
Creatinine	375 µmol/L	70–120 µmol/L
Bicarbonate	18 mmol/L	24–30 mmol/L
Glucose	4.5 mmol/L	4.0–6.0 mmol/L

Urinalysis: –< protein; – blood

Questions

- What are the potential causes of this patient's renal failure?
- How would you investigate and manage this patient?

ANSWER 100

This woman has significant renal failure with associated acidosis and anaemia. Her urinalysis is negative, which excludes a glomerular disease. It is more likely that her renal failure is due to either tubulointerstitial disease or disease affecting the renal vasculature such as accelerated phase hypertension. Potential causes of tubulointerstitial disease in this case are the NSAIDs and the herbal medicines. Her hypertension is likely secondary to her tubulointerstitial disease, and is accelerating the progression of her renal failure.

NSAIDs cause acute kidney injury by two different mechanisms: haemodyamically mediated and acute interstitial nephritis. Haemodynamically mediated acute renal failure is due to inhibition of prostaglandin synthesis. Prostaglandins cause prerenal vasodilatation which is crucial to maintain renal perfusion in the setting of hypovolaemia, cirrhosis and heart failure. In this case there is no evidence that she Is dehydrated. NSAIDs also cause an acute interstitial nephritis. There may be an associated fever, rash, eosinophilia and eosinophiluria. Spontaneous recovery occurs within a few months after the NSAID is discontinued although there may be permanent renal damage. A course of prednisolone is generally given to accelerate renal recovery and lessen long-term scarring. NSAIDs can also induce minimal change disease and membranous nephropathy causing nephritic syndrome. In addition to these acute effects, it has been suggested that daily NSAID use for a prolonged period of time may be associated with an increased risk of chronic kidney disease, although the percentage of patients is small relative to the number of NSAIDs that are bought over the counter.

Traditional Chinese medicine includes herbal therapy, acupuncture, massage and dietary therapy. There is potential for developing novel treatments for diseases such as asthma and food allergies with Chinese herbs. However, there is concern over the lack of standardization and controlled clinical trials. Chinese herbal medicines containing aristolochic acid have been implicated in a specific nephropathy characterised by extensive interstitial fibrosis with atrophy and loss of the tubules, with thickening of the walls of the interlobular and afferent arterioles. Blood pressure is generally normal or only modestly elevated. Patients presenting with a creatinine < 200 will generally stabilise their renal function after stopping the Chinese medications, but patients with worse kidney function will generally progress to end-stage kidney failure.

In this case it is important to find out if her renal failure is acute or long-standing. This can easily be discovered if she has had previous measurements of her serum creatinine. Renal ultrasound is also helpful. If the ultrasound shows small echogenic kidneys her renal failure is likely chronic. If her kidneys are normal in size, a renal biopsy is indicated to confirm the diagnosis and assess the extent of inflammation and scarring.

In this case her renal failure is likely due to a NSAID-induced interstitial nephritis. She should be advised to stop her NSAIDs and Chinese herbal medicines, and never to restart these drugs. She should be given a short course of prednisolone to hasten renal recovery.

 KEY POINTS

- A full drug history is vital in patients with unexplained renal failure.
- NSAIDs are the commonest drug implicated in acute interstitial nephritis.
- Aristolochic acid–containing Chinese herbal medicines cause a characteristic nephropathy.

INDEX

References are by case number with relevant page number(s) following in brackets. References with a page range e.g. 25(68–70) indicate that although the subject may be mentioned on only one page, it concerns the whole case.

DATE DUE
